PROSTATE HEALTH

A Doctor's Practical Guide to Early detection & Care

Dr Prabhat Das

MD, PhD, FACP

Better Health with Dr Das Series

Hardcover ISBN: 978-1-971672-55-7

Paperback ISBN: 978-1-971672-54-0

eBook ISBN: 978-1-971672-53-3

Printed in the United States of America

Disclaimer

This book is intended solely for educational and informational purposes. It is not meant to replace personal medical advice, diagnosis, or treatment.

Although I am a licensed physician, reading this book does not establish a doctor-patient relationship. Each individual's health condition, medical history, and risk factors are unique. Any medical decision should be made in partnership with your own healthcare professional who understands your specific situation.

Medical science is continually advancing. New research and updated guidelines may lead to changes in recommendations over time.

TABLE OF CONTENTS:

About the Author

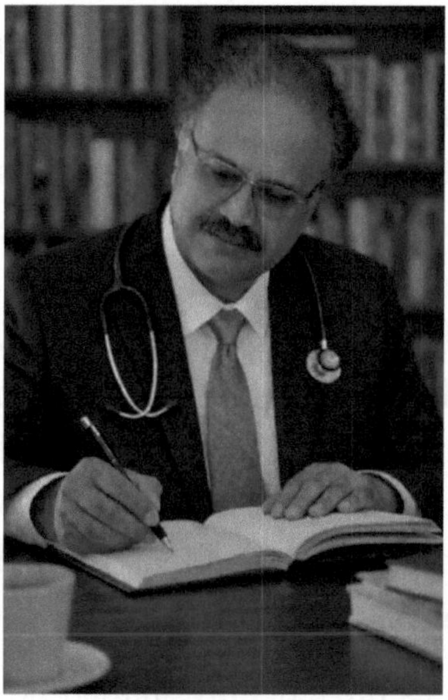

I am Dr Prabhat Das, MD, PhD, FACP. My journey in medicine began in India and, over the past thirty-five years, has continued in the United States, where I have had the privilege of caring for patients across a wide range of medical settings. I am trained in Internal Medicine, Pulmonary Diseases, and Critical Care. For me, medicine has never been just a profession. It has been a lifelong commitment shaped by learning, service, and a deep respect for the trust patients place in their physician.

Over the years, I have had the honor of caring for patients in many different situations. I have seen individuals in my office for routine concerns, treated urgent conditions in busy emergency rooms, managed serious illnesses in the hospital, and cared for critically ill patients in intensive care units. Each setting has taught me something valuable. Each patient has added to my understanding of what it truly means to care for another human being.

But one lesson has stood above all others. Medicine is not only about tests, diagnoses, or treatments. It is about people. It is about listening carefully, understanding fears that are often left unspoken, and guiding patients through uncertainty with clarity and compassion. Again and again, I have seen that what people want most is simple, trustworthy information. They want to understand what is happening in their bodies. They want to feel confident about the decisions they are making for their health and for their families.

These experiences have deeply shaped how I think about health, illness, prevention, and the human side of healing.

That is the reason behind the '**Better Health with Dr Das Series**'. Through these books, I hope to reach individuals I may never meet in person but who are searching for clear and reliable guidance. In today's world, health information is everywhere, yet much of it is confusing, overwhelming, and sometimes misleading. My goal is to cut through that noise and present important medical topics in a way that is simple, practical, and reassuring.

Every page of this series is guided by two foundations: reliable scientific knowledge and decades of real-world clinical experience. I want you, the reader, to feel informed, confident, and empowered. Not overwhelmed. Not confused. But clear about what you can do, step by step, to improve your health.

If even one reader feels less anxious, more informed, or better prepared to take control of their health after reading these books, then this work has served its purpose.

Helping people live healthier, longer, more confident and better-informed lives remains one of the greatest privileges of my life.

CHAPTER 1: Why Every Man Should Understand His Prostate

A Quiet Beginning That Deserves Attention

For most of a man's life, the prostate remains unnoticed.

It does its job quietly, without pain, without warning, without demanding attention. In younger years, there is no reason to think about it. Life moves forward with work, responsibilities, family, and the usual rhythm of daily living.

Then, slowly, almost gently, something begins to change.

You may notice that your urine stream is not as strong as before. It may take a little longer. You may wake up once at night, then again a few months later, and gradually it becomes part of your routine. You adjust without thinking much about it.

Many men say the same thing.

"This is just aging."

There is some truth in that. But it is not the full story.

Aging is natural. Quietly accepting discomfort is not necessary.

Why This Topic Matters More Than You Think

Prostate-related symptoms are among the most common health concerns in men after the age of 40 or 50.

At first, they may seem minor. A little inconvenience. A small disturbance in routine.

But over time, they begin to affect:

- Sleep
- Energy
- Daily comfort
- Confidence
- Peace of mind

And sometimes, they raise a deeper concern.

"Could this be something serious?"

That question, more than the symptom itself, is what troubles most men.

The Fear That Needs to Be Addressed

For many, the word "prostate" immediately brings one thought.

Cancer.

That fear is understandable. But it is often misplaced or exaggerated.

Let me say something very clearly at the beginning of this book.

Most prostate problems are not cancer.

Many are due to simple enlargement or temporary inflammation. Even when cancer is present, it does not always behave aggressively. In fact, many prostate cancers grow slowly and can be managed effectively.

Fear without understanding leads to two common mistakes:

- Ignoring symptoms completely
- Panicking over small findings

Neither helps.

Understanding changes everything.

The Three Conditions Every Man Should Know

Almost all prostate-related concerns fall into three main categories.

- Enlarged prostate, also called benign prostatic hyperplasia
- Prostatitis, which is inflammation

- Prostate cancer

Each of these behaves differently. Each requires a different approach.

But here is where confusion begins.

The symptoms can overlap.

That is why guessing is not helpful. A clear understanding is.

Why Men Often Delay Getting Help

Over the years, I have seen a pattern.

Men tend to wait.

They wait because:

- Symptoms seem mild
- They feel embarrassed discussing urinary or sexual issues
- They assume it is part of aging
- They fear what the diagnosis might reveal

This delay is rarely helpful.

In most cases, earlier evaluation leads to simpler solutions and better outcomes.

Seeking help is not a sign of weakness. It is a sign of awareness.

What This Book Will Do for You

This book is not written as a medical textbook.

It is written the way I speak to my patients.

Simple. Clear. Practical.

My goal is to help you:

- Understand what the prostate does
- Recognize symptoms early
- Understand tests like PSA without fear
- Know when to act and when to observe
- Make informed decisions about treatment
- Protect your long-term health

This is not just about disease.

It is about **confidence, clarity, and control over your health**.

A Small Change in Thinking

Instead of asking:

"What if something is wrong?"

Try asking:

"What is my body trying to tell me?"

This small shift changes everything.

You move from fear to awareness.

From avoidance to action.

A Reflection From Practice

I remember a gentleman in his late fifties.

He had mild symptoms for years. He ignored them. Adjusted his routine. Woke up multiple times at night but never mentioned it during routine visits.

One day, he finally brought it up.

His condition was simple. Easily manageable.

But what stayed with me was what he said later.

"I wish I had asked earlier."

That sentence is the reason this book exists.

Doctor's Pearl

Most prostate problems are manageable when understood early. The real problem is not the condition itself, but the delay in recognizing and addressing it.

CHAPTER 1

THE PROSTATE: BASICS YOU NEED TO UNDERSTAND

The prostate is a small gland in men that plays an important role in the urinary and reproductive systems.

THE MALE URINARY SYSTEM

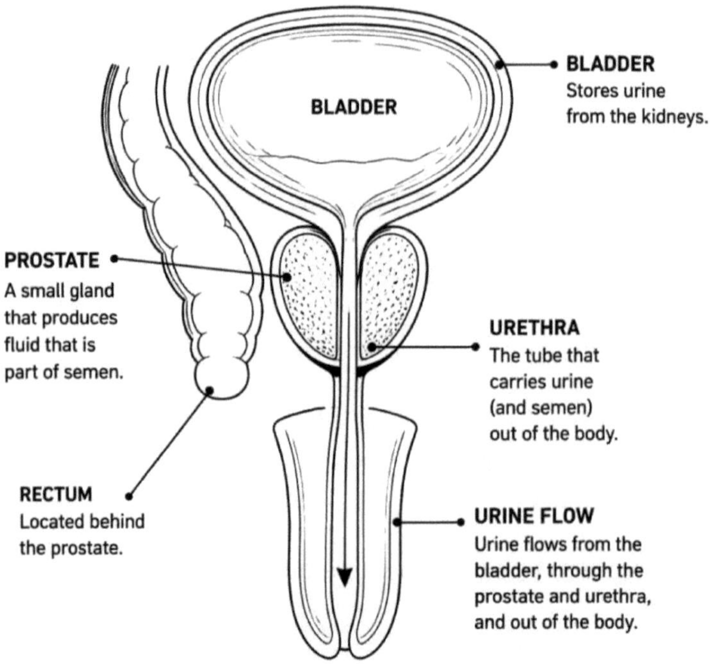

KEY TAKEAWAY

The prostate surrounds the urethra.
When the prostate enlarges or becomes inflamed, it can affect urine flow and cause symptoms.

Chapter Summary

- The prostate is often ignored until symptoms appear
- Urinary symptoms are common but should not be dismissed
- Most prostate problems are not cancer
- Fear and misunderstanding lead to delay
- Early awareness leads to better outcomes
- Understanding your body is the first step toward better health

---

Action Plan

- Begin paying attention to your urinary habits
- Notice changes in flow, frequency, and night-time urination
- Do not ignore persistent symptoms
- Avoid unnecessary fear, but stay aware
- Be open to discussing concerns with your doctor

Moving Forward

You have taken the first and most important step.

Awareness.

In the next chapter, we will build on this foundation. I will help you understand the prostate in simple, clear terms, so that everything you read afterward makes complete sense.

Once you understand the structure, the rest becomes easy.

Let us move forward, step by step.

CHAPTER 2: The Prostate Explained in Plain English

A Simple Picture That Explains Everything

Before we talk about diseases, tests, or treatments, we need a clear picture in the mind.

The prostate is a small gland, about the size of a walnut in younger men. It sits just below the bladder. The tube that carries urine out of the body, the urethra, passes directly through the center of the prostate.

That one fact explains most prostate problems.

If the prostate changes in size or structure, it can affect the flow of urine.

I often tell my patients to imagine a soft ring around a pipe. If the ring thickens or tightens, the flow through the pipe becomes slower. That is exactly what happens when the prostate enlarges.

Once you see this picture clearly, many symptoms begin to make sense.

What Does the Prostate Actually Do?

The prostate plays a role in reproduction.

It produces a fluid that mixes with sperm to form semen. This fluid helps nourish and transport sperm.

That is its biological role.

But from a practical point of view, there is something important to understand.

A man can live a full, healthy, active life even if the prostate is not functioning normally, or even if it has been treated or removed for medical reasons.

This understanding becomes very helpful later, when we discuss treatment. It reduces unnecessary fear.

Why the Prostate Changes With Age

One of the most important facts about the prostate is this.

It tends to grow as men get older.

This growth is influenced by male hormones, especially testosterone and its related forms. Over time, these hormonal effects lead to gradual enlargement of prostate tissue.

This is a natural process.

Many men develop some degree of enlargement with age. Some notice symptoms. Others do not.

This condition is called benign prostatic hyperplasia, or BPH.

Let me make this very clear.

BPH is not cancer. It does not turn into cancer.

It is simply an age-related change.

How These Changes Affect Urination

Because the urethra passes through the prostate, even a small increase in size can affect urine flow.

This can lead to:

- A weaker stream
- Difficulty starting urination
- A feeling of incomplete emptying
- More frequent urination

At the same time, the bladder also responds.

When it has to push harder against resistance, it becomes more sensitive. This leads to urgency and frequent trips to the bathroom.

So the problem is not only in the prostate. It is also in how the bladder reacts.

CHAPTER 2

HOW ENLARGED PROSTATE BLOCKS URINE FLOW

As the prostate enlarges, it squeezes the urethra and makes it harder for urine to pass.

NORMAL PROSTATE

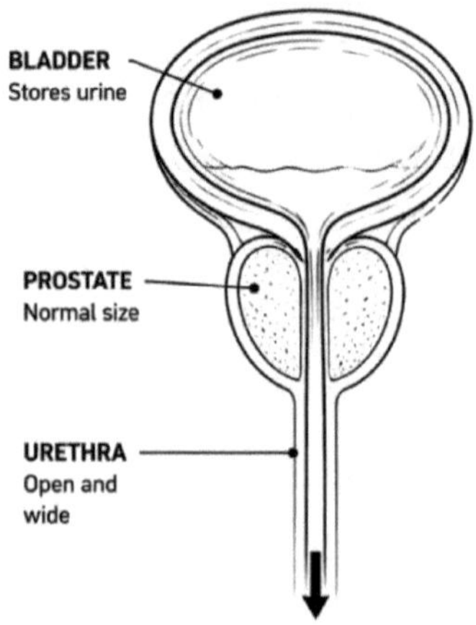

NORMAL FLOW
Urine flows easily through the open urethra.

ENLARGED PROSTATE (BPH)

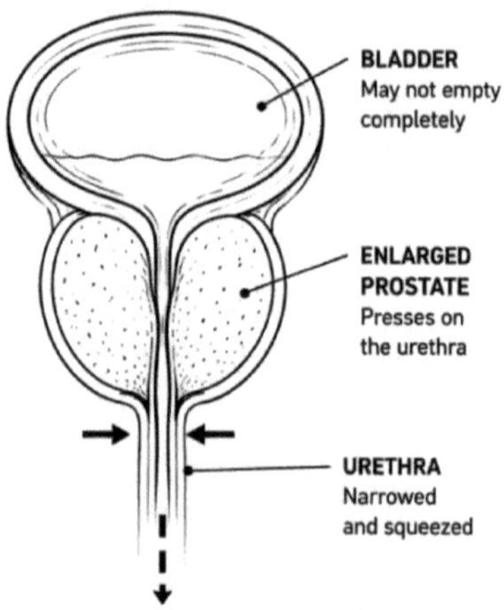

BLOCKED FLOW
Urine flow is restricted, weak, or interrupted.

WHAT HAPPENS OVER TIME?

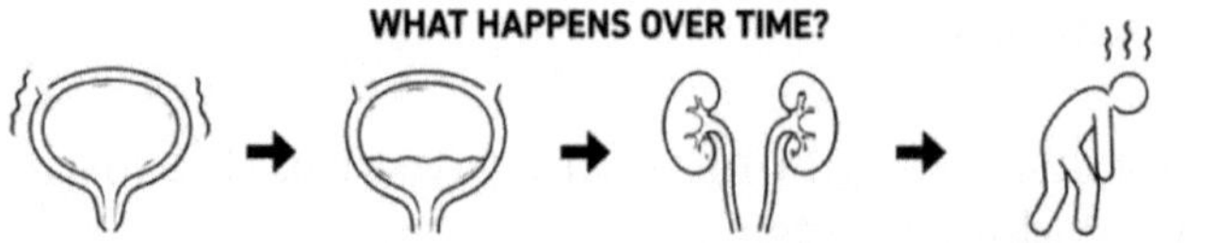

1. Bladder works harder to push urine out.
2. Bladder may not empty completely.
3. Pressure can affect the kidneys in severe cases.
4. Leads to symptoms and reduced quality of life.

KEY TAKEAWAY

An enlarged prostate narrows the urethra, making it difficult to pass urine. Early attention can prevent complications and improve quality of life.

The Prostate, Bladder, and Kidneys Work as a Team

It helps to think of the urinary system as a coordinated system.

The kidneys produce urine.
The bladder stores urine.
The prostate surrounds the outlet.
The urethra carries urine out.

When the prostate begins to narrow the outlet, the entire system adjusts.

The bladder works harder. Over time, this can lead to changes in how it functions.

In more advanced situations, pressure can even affect the kidneys.

This is not common early on, but it reminds us why symptoms should not be ignored for too long.

A Simple Everyday Analogy

Let me make this even simpler.

Imagine a water tank connected to a pipe.

The tank is your bladder.
The pipe is your urethra.
The prostate is like a clamp around that pipe.

If the clamp tightens, the flow slows down. The tank has to push harder. Over time, the system becomes strained.

This simple picture explains most prostate-related urinary problems.

What This Means for You

You do not need to remember complex medical terms.

What matters is understanding this basic relationship.

The prostate sits in a very important position. When it changes, you feel the effects in your daily life, especially in your urination pattern.

Once you understand this, you are no longer guessing. You are observing with awareness.

Doctor's Pearl

Do not focus only on how big the prostate is. What matters most is how it affects urine flow and your quality of life.

Chapter Summary

- The prostate is a small gland located below the bladder

- The urethra passes through it, making it important for urine flow
- Its main function is to contribute fluid to semen
- The prostate commonly enlarges with age
- Enlargement can affect urination and bladder behavior
- Understanding this simple structure makes all prostate problems easier to understand

---

Action Plan

- Visualize the prostate as a ring around the urinary channel
- Connect your symptoms to this simple structure
- Do not assume enlargement is dangerous
- Pay attention to gradual changes in urination
- Keep this basic understanding in mind as you move forward

Now that you clearly understand what the prostate is and how it works, the next step is to understand what can go wrong.

In the next chapter, we will look at the three main prostate conditions side by side, so you can clearly see how they differ and why proper evaluation is important.

CHAPTER 3: The Three Prostate Problems Every Man Should Understand

Clarity Removes Fear

By now, you have a clear picture of where the prostate sits and how it affects urine flow.

The next step is to understand what can go wrong.

Most men do not walk into a clinic with a diagnosis. They come with symptoms. A weak stream, frequent urination, discomfort, or worry after a blood test.

The challenge is simple.

The same symptoms can come from different conditions.

If you understand the three main prostate problems, you will feel more in control. You will know what is common, what needs attention, and what questions to ask.

The Three Conditions That Matter Most

Almost all prostate-related issues fall into three groups:

- Enlarged prostate, also called benign prostatic hyperplasia or BPH

- Prostatitis, which means inflammation of the prostate
- Prostate cancer

Each behaves differently. Each needs a different approach.

Enlarged Prostate (BPH): Common and Manageable

This is the most common condition.

As men age, the prostate tends to grow. This growth is not cancer. It does not spread to other parts of the body. It is a benign process.

However, because the prostate surrounds the urethra, enlargement can narrow the urinary passage.

Typical symptoms include:

- Weak or slow urine stream
- Difficulty starting urination
- Frequent urination
- Waking up at night to urinate
- Feeling that the bladder is not completely empty

These symptoms usually develop gradually.

Many men live with BPH for years. With proper care, symptoms can be controlled, and life can remain comfortable.

UNDERSTANDING SYMPTOMS

Flow Symptoms vs Storage Symptoms

Symptoms of prostate problems can be grouped into two main types. Knowing the difference helps in proper evaluation and treatment.

FLOW SYMPTOMS (Voiding Symptoms)

These symptoms occur while you are urinating.

Weak urine stream
Urine comes out slowly or with low pressure.

Difficulty starting urination
Takes time or effort to get urine started.

Stopping and starting
Urine flow pauses and starts repeatedly.

Feeling of incomplete emptying
Feeling that the bladder is not fully empty.

Dribbling after urination
Small drops of urine leak after finishing.

STORAGE SYMPTOMS (Irritative Symptoms)

These symptoms occur when the bladder is filling.

Urgency
A sudden, strong need to pass urine.

Frequent urination
Needing to pass urine more often than usual.

Nighttime urination
Waking up one or more times at night to urinate.

Small volume each time
Passing only a small amount of urine.

Urge incontinence
Leakage of urine when you cannot reach the toilet in time.

HOW THEY AFFECT YOUR DAILY LIFE

Poor sleep | Fatigue | Discomfort | Social limitation | Reduced quality of life

KEY TAKEAWAY

Identifying whether your symptoms are related to urine flow or storage helps your doctor find the right cause and treatment for you.

Prostatitis: When Discomfort Takes the Lead

Prostatitis is different.

It is not about size. It is about inflammation.

Sometimes it is caused by infection. Sometimes no infection is found. In many cases, it behaves like a chronic pain condition.

Symptoms often include:

- Burning during urination
- Pain in the lower abdomen, pelvis, or back
- Discomfort during or after ejaculation
- Frequent or urgent urination

This condition can affect younger men as well.

One of the most frustrating aspects is that symptoms may come and go. Tests may appear normal. That does not mean the problem is not real.

Prostate Cancer: Important, But Not Always Urgent

Prostate cancer is the condition that creates the most concern.

It is important to understand it correctly.

Some prostate cancers grow very slowly and may never cause harm. Others are more aggressive and need timely treatment.

In early stages, prostate cancer often causes no symptoms. That is why it is sometimes detected through PSA testing.

When symptoms do appear, they may include:

- Difficulty urinating
- Blood in urine
- Bone pain in advanced stages

But these are usually later signs.

The key message is this.

A diagnosis of prostate cancer is not always an emergency. It requires careful evaluation.

Why These Conditions Feel Similar

This is where confusion begins.

All three conditions can affect urination.

You may have a weak stream, frequency, or urgency in any of them.

That is why symptoms alone cannot give a diagnosis.

Proper evaluation is necessary.

When You Should Be More Alert

Most symptoms are not emergencies, but some signs should prompt quicker attention:

- Blood in urine or semen
- Severe pain with fever
- Sudden inability to pass urine
- Unexplained weight loss
- Persistent bone pain

These symptoms do not always mean something serious, but they should never be ignored.

A Simple Way to Remember

If you want to keep things clear in your mind:

- BPH is mainly about enlargement
- Prostatitis is mainly about inflammation
- Cancer is about abnormal cell growth

This simple framework helps reduce confusion.

A Reflection From Practice

A man in his early sixties came to me with urinary symptoms. He was convinced he had cancer.

After proper evaluation, his condition turned out to be simple prostate enlargement.

With treatment, his symptoms improved, and his fear disappeared.

His biggest problem was not the prostate. It was uncertainty.

Doctor's Pearl

Most prostate symptoms are caused by non-cancerous conditions. Do not assume the worst, but do not ignore symptoms either.

Chapter Summary

- The three main prostate conditions are BPH, prostatitis, and prostate cancer
- BPH is common and non-cancerous
- Prostatitis often causes discomfort and pain
- Prostate cancer varies widely in behavior
- Symptoms can overlap and require proper evaluation
- Certain warning signs need prompt medical attention

Action Plan

- Stay calm when symptoms appear
- Look at the pattern of symptoms, not just one change
- Seek medical advice if symptoms persist
- Pay attention to warning signs
- Maintain a balanced and informed approach

Now that you understand the three main prostate conditions, the next step is to recognize how they show up in everyday life.

In the next chapter, we will look closely at urinary symptoms, so you can clearly understand what your body is trying to tell you.

CHAPTER 4: Urinary Symptoms Men Should Not Ignore

Learning to Listen to Your Body

Most prostate problems do not announce themselves loudly.

They begin quietly. A small change here, a slight inconvenience there.

A weaker stream. A little hesitation. One extra visit to the bathroom at night.

It is easy to ignore these changes. Life is busy, and we adapt. Many men simply adjust their routine and move on.

But the body has its own language.

Symptoms are signals. When you learn to recognize them early, you gain control. When you ignore them for too long, they slowly begin to control you.

The Common Symptoms You May Notice

Let us go through the symptoms that many men experience.

Weak urine stream
The flow is not as strong as before. It may take longer to finish.

Hesitation
You are ready to urinate, but it takes time to start.

Intermittent flow
The stream may stop and start during urination.

Frequency
You feel the need to urinate more often than usual.

Urgency
A sudden need to urinate that is difficult to delay.

Nocturia
Waking up at night to urinate. Once may be manageable. Repeated awakenings disturb sleep.

Incomplete emptying
A feeling that the bladder is not fully empty even after urination.

Each of these may seem small, but together they can affect daily comfort in a significant way.

Understanding Flow and Storage Symptoms

To make sense of these changes, it helps to group them.

Flow symptoms
These are related to difficulty passing urine:

- Weak stream
- Hesitation
- Straining
- Interrupted flow

These often suggest some blockage at the level of the prostate.

Storage symptoms
These are related to how the bladder behaves:

- Frequency
- Urgency
- Night-time urination

These often indicate that the bladder has become more sensitive or overactive.

Most men have a mix of both.

How Symptoms Affect Daily Life

At first, symptoms are an inconvenience.

Over time, they begin to shape your routine.

You may start planning your day around restroom access.
Long drives may feel uncomfortable.
Meetings may feel longer than they should.
Sleep becomes interrupted.

Gradually, this leads to:

- Fatigue
- Reduced concentration
- Irritability

These are not minor issues. They affect your quality of life.

When Pain Is Present

Pain is an important signal.

If you notice:

- Burning during urination
- Pain in the lower abdomen or pelvic area
- Discomfort during or after ejaculation

This often points toward inflammation, such as prostatitis.

Pain should always be evaluated. It is the body asking for attention.

Red Flag Warnings

Some symptoms require prompt medical attention.

These include:

- Blood in urine or semen
- Sudden inability to urinate

- Fever along with urinary symptoms
- Severe pelvic or back pain
- Unexplained weight loss

These do not always mean something serious, but they should never be ignored.

A Reflection From Practice

A gentleman once told me, “Doctor, I have arranged my life around the bathroom.”

He was waking up multiple times at night and avoiding long outings.

He had accepted this as normal.

After evaluation and treatment, his symptoms improved significantly. His sleep improved. His energy returned.

What surprised him most was not the treatment.

It was how much better he could feel.

Doctor’s Pearl

Symptoms are early signals. Recognizing them early often makes treatment simpler and more effective.

Chapter Summary

- Urinary symptoms are often the first sign of prostate problems
- Common symptoms include weak stream, urgency, and night-time urination
- Symptoms can be grouped into flow and storage types
- These changes gradually affect daily life and sleep
- Pain suggests inflammation and needs attention
- Certain warning signs require prompt evaluation

Action Plan

- Pay attention to changes in your urination pattern
- Keep track of how often you wake up at night
- Do not ignore persistent or worsening symptoms
- Seek medical advice when symptoms affect your daily life
- Stay calm, but stay aware

Now that you can recognize symptoms clearly, the next step is to understand how these symptoms affect your overall health.

In the next chapter, we will look beyond the urinary system and understand how prostate problems can influence sleep, energy, kidneys, and overall well-being.

CHAPTER 5: How Prostate Problems Affect Your Whole Body

It Is Never Just About Urination

When most men think about prostate problems, they think about the bathroom.

How often they go. How strong the stream is. How many times they wake up at night.

But in real life, prostate problems rarely stay limited to urination.

Over time, they begin to affect the whole person.

Sleep changes. Energy declines. Mood shifts. Confidence is affected. Even relationships may feel different.

This chapter is about seeing that larger picture.

The Bladder Under Constant Strain

Let us begin with the bladder.

When the prostate narrows the urinary passage, the bladder has to work harder to push urine out.

In the early stages, it adapts well. The muscle becomes stronger and pushes with more force.

But this constant effort cannot continue forever.

Over time, the bladder may:

- Become overactive, leading to urgency and frequency
- Become thickened due to constant strain
- Lose efficiency, leading to incomplete emptying

This is why some men feel the need to urinate again soon after they have just finished.

The issue is no longer only the prostate. The bladder is now involved.

Sleep: The First Silent Casualty

Sleep is often the first major area to suffer.

Waking up once at night may not seem important.

But waking up three or four times every night gradually changes how you feel during the day.

Over weeks and months, this leads to:

- Daytime fatigue
- Reduced concentration
- Irritability
- Lower productivity

Many men do not connect their tiredness to their urinary symptoms.

But once the night-time urination improves, their energy often returns.

Energy, Mood, and Daily Function

When sleep is disturbed, everything else follows.

You may notice:

- Less energy for daily activities
- Reduced interest in exercise
- Increased frustration over small things
- Difficulty focusing

These are not separate problems.

They are part of the same chain reaction that begins with repeated interruptions during the night.

Kidneys: Rarely Affected, But Important

The kidneys quietly filter blood and produce urine.

In most early prostate problems, they remain unaffected.

But in advanced cases, when urine cannot flow properly for a long time, pressure can build up backward toward the kidneys.

This can interfere with normal kidney function.

This is not common, but when it happens, it becomes serious.

The important message is simple.

Early attention prevents these complications.

Sexual Health and Confidence

Prostate problems can influence sexual health in several ways.

Some men notice changes in erections. Others feel discomfort during ejaculation. Many feel less confident because of ongoing symptoms.

Even when physical changes are mild, the emotional impact can be significant.

Confidence plays a major role in sexual health.

When a man feels uncertain about his body, it affects his sense of well-being.

EFFECTS OF PROSTATE PROBLEMS ON YOUR BODY

Prostate problems can affect more than just urination. They can impact your daily life and overall well-being.

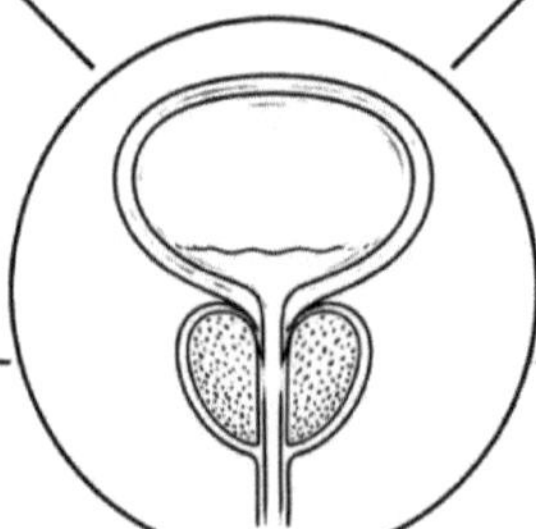

SLEEP DISTURBANCE

- Frequent nighttime urination
- Poor sleep quality
- Daytime tiredness

BLADDER EFFECTS

- Incomplete emptying
- Overactive bladder
- Increased bladder pressure

KIDNEY IMPACT

- Back pressure can affect kidneys
- May cause kidney damage over time
- Can lead to infections

SEXUAL HEALTH

- Reduced sexual desire
- Erectile difficulties
- Ejaculatory problems

INFECTION RISK

- Stagnant urine can increase infections
- May cause burning, pain and fever

MENTAL WELL-BEING

- Worry and stress
- Anxiety about symptoms
- Reduced confidence and mood

OVERALL QUALITY OF LIFE

- Limits daily activities
- Affects work and productivity
- Reduces enjoyment of life

KEY TAKEAWAY

Prostate problems can affect many parts of your body and life. Early attention, proper treatment and healthy habits can help protect your overall health and well-being.

The Emotional Burden of Ongoing Symptoms

Living with persistent symptoms has a psychological impact.

You may find yourself:

- Planning your day around restroom access
- Avoiding long trips
- Feeling concerned about your health
- Becoming more anxious than before

These changes often happen gradually.

Many men accept them without realizing how much their quality of life has changed.

How Life Slowly Adjusts Without You Noticing

Prostate symptoms rarely create a sudden crisis.

Instead, they quietly reshape your routine.

You wake up tired.
You adjust your activities.
You limit certain situations.
You become more cautious.

This gradual change becomes your new normal.

But it does not have to be.

A Reflection From Practice

A patient once came to me complaining mainly of low energy.

He thought he needed vitamins or some form of general treatment.

During our discussion, he mentioned waking up multiple times at night to urinate.

We focused on his urinary symptoms.

As his night-time urination improved, his energy returned.

The solution was not complicated. It was simply understanding the real cause.

Doctor's Pearl

When a small symptom continues for a long time, it can create a large impact. Never underestimate the effect of repeated night-time urination.

Chapter Summary

- Prostate problems affect more than urination
- The bladder can become overworked and less efficient
- Sleep disturbance is a major consequence

- Energy and mood are closely linked to sleep quality
- Kidney involvement is rare but possible in advanced cases
- Sexual health and confidence may be affected
- Quality of life gradually declines when symptoms are ignored

---

Action Plan

- Notice how symptoms affect your sleep and energy
- Do not ignore frequent night-time urination
- Pay attention to both physical and emotional changes
- Seek help early rather than adjusting silently
- Remember that improvement is possible with proper care

Now that you understand the broader impact of prostate problems, the next step is to understand what can happen if these issues are ignored.

In the next chapter, we will discuss possible complications and why timely action makes a meaningful difference.

CHAPTER 6: What Can Happen If Prostate Problems Are Ignored

The Hidden Cost of “I’ll Wait and See”

Many men are patient with their health.

“I’ll give it some time.”
“It is not too bad yet.”
“It will settle on its own.”

Sometimes that approach works. But with prostate problems, it often leads to a slow buildup of avoidable trouble.

Let me be clear from the start.

Prostate conditions usually do not become dangerous overnight. They progress gradually. That is exactly why they are easy to ignore.

But gradual does not mean harmless.

The Bladder Works Harder Than It Should

In the early stage, the bladder compensates.

It pushes harder to empty urine through a narrowed passage. For a while, it manages.

Over time, that extra effort begins to show.

The bladder may:

- Become overactive, leading to urgency and frequency
- Become thickened from constant strain
- Lose strength, leading to incomplete emptying

This is when men start to feel that the bladder never truly empties.

A small amount of urine remains behind. This is called residual urine, and it sets the stage for further problems.

Acute Urinary Retention: When It Becomes an Emergency

One of the most uncomfortable situations is sudden inability to pass urine.

This is called acute urinary retention.

The bladder becomes painfully full. There is pressure, discomfort, and often anxiety. It requires urgent medical attention.

A catheter is usually needed to relieve the bladder.

Many men who experience this had symptoms for months or years but delayed seeking care.

A manageable problem becomes an emergency simply because it was ignored.

Repeated Infections

When urine remains in the bladder, bacteria find an opportunity to grow.

This can lead to repeated urinary infections.

You may notice:

- Burning during urination
- Fever
- Cloudy or foul-smelling urine

These infections can recur and become a repeated source of discomfort.

Long-Term Bladder Damage

Chronic strain changes the structure of the bladder.

The wall becomes thick and less flexible. Small outpouchings may develop. Over time, the bladder may lose its ability to contract properly.

At this stage, even if the prostate problem is treated, the bladder may not fully recover.

This is why timing matters.

Effects on the Kidneys

In advanced cases, pressure from the bladder can travel upward.

This can affect how urine drains from the kidneys.

Over time, this may impact kidney function.

This is not common in early stages, but when it occurs, it becomes serious.

The important point is this.

These complications are often preventable with early care.

When Prostate Cancer Progresses Quietly

Prostate cancer behaves differently.

In its early stages, it may not cause any symptoms at all.

That means a man may feel completely well while the disease is present.

If not detected and monitored, some cancers can progress.

Later signs may include:

- Persistent bone pain
- Unexplained weight loss
- Fatigue

Not all cancers behave this way, but some do.

Early detection provides more choices and better outcomes.

The Emotional Burden of Ongoing Symptoms

There is another cost that is often overlooked.

Living with ongoing symptoms slowly affects how you feel.

You may experience:

- Tiredness due to poor sleep
- Frustration from repeated interruptions
- Concern about your health
- Reduced confidence in daily activities

These changes are gradual but meaningful.

A Reflection From Practice

A man in his mid-sixties came to the emergency room with acute urinary retention.

He had ignored symptoms for years.

By the time he sought help, his bladder had already been affected.

After treatment, he said something that stayed with me.

“I should have come earlier.”

That is a sentence I have heard many times.

Doctor’s Pearl

Most prostate problems are manageable when addressed early. Delay does not make them disappear. It only makes them harder to treat.

Chapter Summary

- Prostate problems often progress slowly but can lead to complications
- The bladder may become overworked and eventually weakened
- Acute urinary retention is a painful emergency
- Residual urine increases the risk of infection
- Long-term pressure can damage the bladder and affect kidney function
- Prostate cancer may progress silently in some cases
- Quality of life declines gradually when symptoms are ignored

---

Action Plan

- Do not ignore persistent urinary symptoms
- Seek evaluation before symptoms become severe
- Pay attention to warning signs such as inability to urinate or fever
- Prioritize regular medical follow-up
- Act early for simpler and more effective treatment

Now that you understand the consequences of delay, the next step is to understand one of the most important tools in prostate care.

In the next chapter, we will discuss PSA testing in a calm and practical way, so you can understand it without fear or confusion.

CHAPTER 7: PSA Testing – Clear Understanding Without Unnecessary Fear

A Simple Test That Creates Complex Emotions

Few medical tests create as much anxiety as the PSA test.

A single number on a report can change how a man feels overnight. Sleep may be disturbed. Thoughts may go straight to the worst possibility.

At the same time, some men avoid the test completely because they are afraid of what it might show.

Both reactions come from the same place.

Uncertainty.

This chapter is meant to remove that uncertainty and replace it with clear understanding.

What PSA Actually Means

PSA stands for prostate-specific antigen.

It is a protein produced by the prostate gland. A small amount normally enters the bloodstream, so every man has a PSA level.

This is important to remember.

PSA is not abnormal. It is a normal part of prostate function.

The test simply measures how much of this protein is present in your blood.

Why PSA Levels Can Increase

Many men believe that PSA rises only because of cancer.

That is not correct.

PSA can increase due to several reasons:

- Natural enlargement of the prostate
- Inflammation or infection
- Recent ejaculation
- Medical procedures involving the prostate or urinary tract
- Normal aging
- Prostate cancer

So an elevated PSA is not a diagnosis. It is a signal.

Think of PSA as an Alert, Not a Conclusion

It helps to think of PSA in a simple way.

PSA is like a warning light.

When it rises, it tells us to look more closely. It does not tell us what the exact problem is.

A higher PSA does not confirm cancer.
A lower PSA does not completely rule it out.

Understanding this reduces unnecessary panic.

Why a Single Value Is Not Enough

Many men focus on one number.

In real practice, what matters more is the trend over time.

A PSA that remains stable over years is usually less concerning.

A PSA that is rising steadily may need closer evaluation.

Doctors often look at patterns rather than isolated results.

What Is Considered "Normal"?

This is one of the most confusing areas.

There is no single normal value that applies to every man.

Age matters. Prostate size matters. Previous values matter.

Traditionally, a PSA below 4 has been used as a general guide. But this is not a strict rule.

The same number may mean different things in different individuals.

False Alarms Are Common

Sometimes PSA rises temporarily.

This may lead to repeat testing or further evaluation.

These situations are known as false positives.

They are one reason why PSA testing needs to be interpreted carefully.

The goal is not to avoid the test, but to use it wisely.

When PSA Needs Closer Attention

Certain patterns deserve more careful evaluation:

- A steadily rising PSA
- A significant increase over a short period
- Abnormal findings on examination
- Strong family history

In these situations, your doctor may recommend additional testing.

UNDERSTANDING PSA

THE SIGNAL, NOT THE DIAGNOSIS

PSA (Prostate-Specific Antigen) is a protein made by the prostate. It can be measured in the blood.

PSA LEVELS

NORMAL RANGE
Generally less than 4.0 ng/mL
(May vary with age)

BORDERLINE RANGE
4.0 – 10.0 ng/mL
Needs careful evaluation

HIGH RANGE
Above 10.0 ng/mL
Requires further assessment

Note: PSA levels vary with age, prostate size and individual factors.

PSA CAN RISE DUE TO

- Enlarged Prostate (BPH)
- Prostatitis (Infection/ Inflammation)
- Prostate Cancer
- Vigorous Exercise
- Medical Procedures (e.g., Biopsy)
- Recent Ejaculation

Important:
A high PSA does not mean cancer.
It is only a signal that needs evaluation.

PSA TELLS US	VS	PSA DOES NOT TELL US
✓ That something in the prostate may need attention		✗ Whether cancer is present or not
✓ Helps in early detection of possible problems		✗ How aggressive the cancer is
✓ Helps in monitoring prostate conditions over time		✗ Whether treatment is needed or not

PSA TREND MATTERS MORE THAN A SINGLE NUMBER

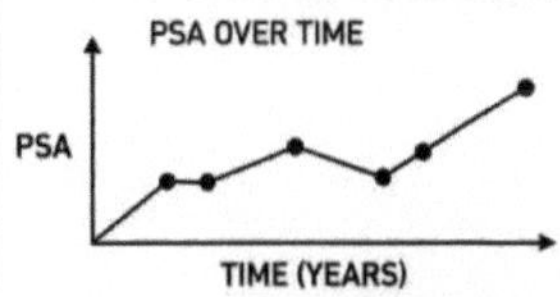

WHAT IT MEANS

- Rising trend: Needs evaluation
- Stable trend: Usually reassuring
- Falling trend: Often a good sign

KEY TAKEAWAY

PSA is a useful tool, but it is not perfect. It should always be interpreted along with age, symptoms, exam and other tests by your doctor.

Myth vs Fact

Myth: A high PSA means cancer
Fact: Many non-cancerous conditions can raise PSA

Myth: A normal PSA means everything is fine
Fact: PSA is helpful but not perfect

Myth: PSA testing always leads to unnecessary treatment
Fact: When used properly, it helps guide appropriate care

A Reflection From Practice

A patient once came to me deeply worried about a small rise in his PSA.

He had already assumed the worst.

When we reviewed his history, the change was minimal and consistent with benign enlargement.

We followed him over time. His PSA remained stable.

His greatest problem was not his prostate. It was fear based on misunderstanding.

Doctor's Pearl

Never interpret a PSA value in isolation. Always look at trends, symptoms, and the overall clinical picture.

Chapter Summary

- PSA is a normal protein produced by the prostate
- Levels can rise due to many non-cancerous reasons
- It is not a definitive test for cancer
- Trends over time are more important than a single value
- Interpretation must be individualized
- Understanding PSA reduces unnecessary anxiety

Action Plan

- Do not panic if your PSA is slightly elevated
- Discuss results carefully with your doctor
- Focus on changes over time rather than one value
- Avoid unnecessary repeated testing without guidance
- Stay informed and balanced

Now that you understand PSA clearly, the next step is to understand how it is used in screening.

In the next chapter, we will discuss prostate cancer screening in a practical and balanced way, so you can decide what is right for you.

CHAPTER 8: Prostate Cancer Screening – A Thoughtful, Personal Decision

Not a Yes or No Answer

Many men ask a direct question.

"Doctor, should I get screened?"

It sounds simple. It is not.

Prostate cancer screening is not a one-size decision. It is a personal choice that depends on your age, your risk, your health, and your comfort with uncertainty.

Two men of the same age may choose different paths, and both can be right.

My role here is not to push you in one direction. It is to help you understand the decision so you can make it with clarity and confidence.

What Screening Means

Screening means looking for disease before symptoms appear.

In prostate health, screening usually involves:

- A PSA blood test
- Sometimes a digital rectal examination

Early prostate cancer often causes no symptoms. Screening can detect it at a stage when more options are available.

What Are the Potential Benefits?

Screening can:

- Detect cancer early
- Increase treatment options
- Improve outcomes in selected men

For men at higher risk, this can be particularly valuable.

Early detection does not guarantee a better outcome in every case, but it often gives more control.

What Are the Limitations?

Screening is not perfect.

It can lead to:

- False alarms, where PSA is elevated but no cancer is present
- Additional testing, including biopsy
- Detection of slow-growing cancers that may never cause harm

This last point is important.

Some prostate cancers are so slow that they would never affect a man's life. Finding them can create anxiety and may lead to treatment that was not truly necessary.

Understanding Overdiagnosis in Simple Terms

Overdiagnosis means finding a condition that would not have caused problems if left undetected.

This can lead to overtreatment.

And treatment, while often effective, can have side effects that affect urination and sexual function.

The goal is balance.

Find the cancers that matter. Avoid unnecessary harm from those that do not.

Who Should Consider Screening?

In general, men between the ages of 50 and 69 benefit from discussing screening with their doctor.

Some men may consider earlier screening:

- Those with a family history of prostate cancer
- Those with known genetic risk

- African American men, who have a higher overall risk

For these groups, earlier and more thoughtful screening may be appropriate.

Who May Not Benefit as Much?

Screening may be less helpful for:

- Men with serious medical conditions
- Men with limited life expectancy
- Very elderly men

In these situations, the risks of testing and follow-up may outweigh the benefits.

Shared Decision-Making: The Right Approach

This is the most important idea in this chapter.

You and your doctor make the decision together.

You consider:

- Your personal risk
- Your values and preferences
- Your willingness to pursue further testing if needed

There is no universal answer. There is only the right answer for you.

Questions That Help You Decide

Before making a decision, ask:

- What is my personal risk?
- What are the benefits in my case?
- What are the possible downsides?
- What happens if my PSA is elevated?

Clear questions lead to clear decisions.

A Reflection From Practice

I remember two patients of similar age.

One chose screening because he wanted early detection under any circumstance.
The other chose to wait because he preferred to avoid unnecessary testing.

Both understood the risks and benefits.

Both were comfortable with their decisions.

That is the goal.

Doctor's Pearl

Screening is not about finding every cancer. It is about finding the cancers that matter, at the right time, in the right person.

Chapter Summary

- Screening aims to detect prostate cancer before symptoms appear
- PSA is the main screening tool
- Screening has both benefits and limitations
- Some detected cancers may never cause harm
- Decisions should be individualized
- Shared discussion with your doctor is essential

Action Plan

- Reflect on your personal risk and preferences
- Discuss screening with your doctor
- Avoid decisions based on fear or avoidance
- Ask clear and practical questions
- Choose a path you understand and are comfortable with

Now that you understand screening, the next step is to understand what happens when you are evaluated.

In the next chapter, we will walk through the diagnostic process step by step, so you know exactly what to expect and why each step is important.

CHAPTER 9: How Prostate Problems Are Diagnosed – A Clear, Step-by-Step Approach

Removing the Fear of the Unknown

For many men, the diagnosis feels more stressful than the symptoms.

"What tests will I need?"
"Will it be painful?"
"Why so many steps?"

These questions are natural.

Let me reassure you.

A good evaluation is not about doing many tests. It is about doing the **right tests, in the right order, for the right reason**.

Once you understand the process, the fear reduces. You know what to expect, and you know why each step matters.

Step 1: A Thoughtful Conversation

Everything begins with listening.

A careful doctor will ask about your symptoms in detail:

- When did they begin?
- How often do you urinate?
- Do you wake up at night?
- Is there pain or burning?
- Do you feel the bladder empties fully?

You may also be asked about:

- Medications
- Past medical history
- Family history

This step is more powerful than it seems. Often, the likely cause becomes clear just from a good conversation.

Step 2: Symptom Scoring – Making It Clear

Doctors may use a simple questionnaire to measure symptoms.

It asks about frequency, urgency, stream, and night-time urination.

Each response is given a score. The total helps classify symptoms as mild, moderate, or severe.

Why this helps:

- It gives a clear starting point
- It allows tracking over time
- It makes discussions more objective

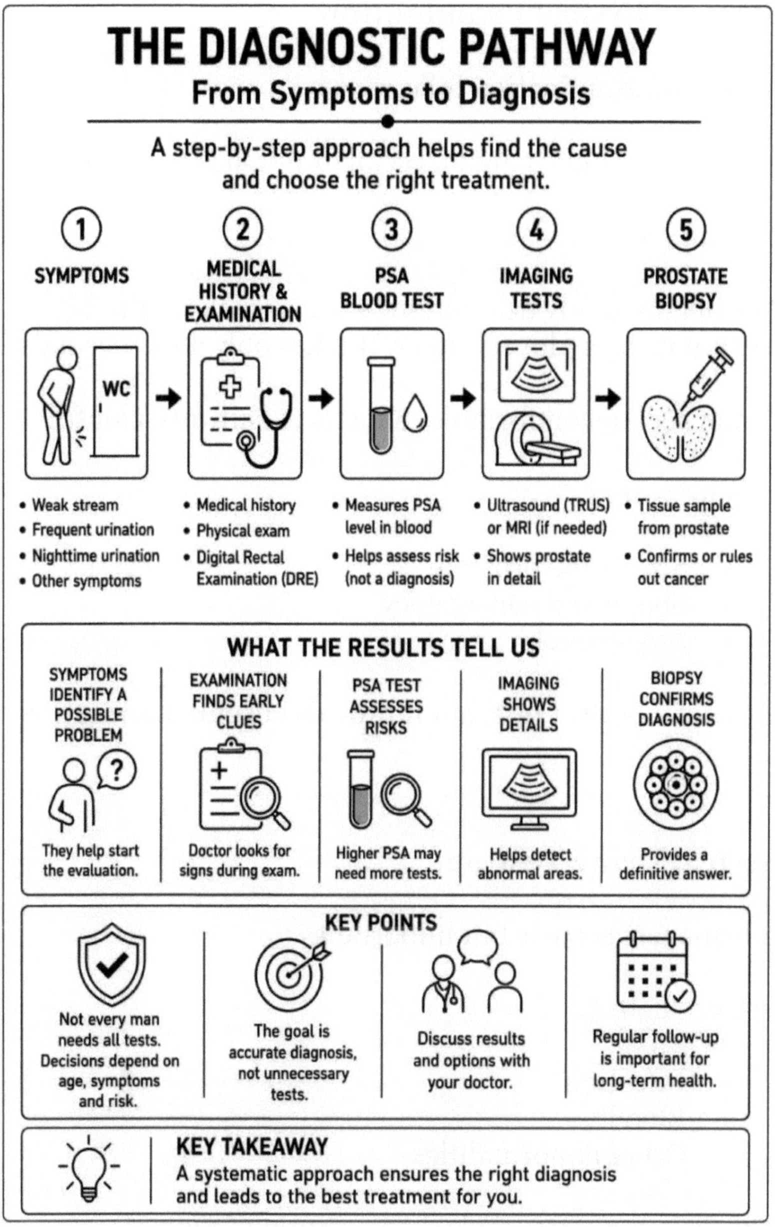
THE DIAGNOSTIC PATHWAY
From Symptoms to Diagnosis
A step-by-step approach helps find the cause and choose the right treatment.
1 SYMPTOMS
2 MEDICAL HISTORY & EXAMINATION
3 PSA BLOOD TEST
4 IMAGING TESTS
5 PROSTATE BIOPSY
WC
• Weak stream
• Frequent urination
• Nighttime urination
• Other symptoms
• Medical history
• Physical exam
• Digital Rectal Examination (DRE)
• Measures PSA level in blood
• Helps assess risk (not a diagnosis)
• Ultrasound (TRUS) or MRI (if needed)
• Shows prostate in detail
• Tissue sample from prostate
• Confirms or rules out cancer
WHAT THE RESULTS TELL US
SYMPTOMS IDENTIFY A POSSIBLE PROBLEM
They help start the evaluation.
EXAMINATION FINDS EARLY CLUES
Doctor looks for signs during exam.
PSA TEST ASSESSES RISKS
Higher PSA may need more tests.
IMAGING SHOWS DETAILS
Helps detect abnormal areas.
BIOPSY CONFIRMS DIAGNOSIS
Provides a definitive answer.
KEY POINTS
Not every man needs all tests. Decisions depend on age, symptoms and risk.
The goal is accurate diagnosis, not unnecessary tests.
Discuss results and options with your doctor.
Regular follow-up is important for long-term health.
KEY TAKEAWAY
A systematic approach ensures the right diagnosis and leads to the best treatment for you.

Step 3: Physical Examination

A focused examination follows.

This may include a digital rectal examination, or DRE.

It is simple.

The doctor gently examines the prostate through the rectum using a gloved finger. It takes only a few seconds.

It may feel uncomfortable, but it is usually not painful.

It helps assess:

- Size of the prostate
- Shape and consistency
- Any irregular areas

It is not a perfect test, but it provides useful information.

Step 4: Urine Testing

A urine test is basic but important.

It helps detect:

- Infection
- Blood
- Other abnormalities

This is especially useful when symptoms suggest inflammation or infection.

Step 5: PSA Blood Test

PSA is one part of the evaluation.

It is interpreted along with:

- Symptoms
- Examination findings
- Age and risk factors

On its own, PSA is just a number. In context, it becomes meaningful.

Step 6: Imaging When Needed

If more clarity is needed, imaging may be used.

Ultrasound

- Measures prostate size
- Checks how well the bladder empties

MRI of the prostate

- Provides detailed images
- Helps identify suspicious areas

MRI has become an important tool, especially when cancer is a concern.

Step 7: Bladder Function Tests

Sometimes the focus shifts to how the bladder is working.

Tests may include:

- Measuring how much urine remains after urination
- Checking the speed of urine flow

These help determine whether symptoms are due to blockage, bladder weakness, or both.

Step 8: Biopsy – Only When Necessary

A biopsy is not done routinely.

It is considered when there is a real concern for cancer.

This may be based on:

- Rising PSA
- Abnormal examination
- Suspicious imaging

Small samples of prostate tissue are taken and examined.

It is an important test, but it is used selectively.

Putting It All Together

No single test gives the full answer.

Diagnosis is based on a combination of:

- Your symptoms
- Physical findings
- Laboratory results
- Imaging when needed

This complete picture guides the next step.

A Reflection From Practice

A man in his early sixties came with frequent urination and a weak stream.

His PSA was slightly elevated, which worried him.

After proper evaluation, imaging showed no concerning findings. His symptoms were due to simple enlargement.

With treatment, he improved without needing invasive procedures.

This is the value of a careful, step-by-step approach.

Doctor's Pearl

Good diagnosis is thoughtful diagnosis. It is not about doing more tests, but about doing the right ones.

Chapter Summary

- Diagnosis begins with a detailed history
- Symptom scoring helps measure severity
- Physical examination provides important clues
- Urine tests detect infection or blood
- PSA adds useful but not definitive information
- Imaging and bladder tests are used when needed
- Biopsy is reserved for specific situations

Action Plan

- Be open and honest about your symptoms
- Do not feel uncomfortable discussing concerns
- Understand that each test has a purpose
- Avoid unnecessary testing without guidance
- Trust a structured, step-by-step evaluation

Now that you understand how prostate problems are diagnosed, we will move to the most common condition affecting men.

In the next chapter, we will take a closer look at enlarged prostate and understand it in a clear, practical, and reassuring way.

CHAPTER 10: Enlarged Prostate (BPH) – Understanding the Most Common Condition in Aging Men

A Natural Change That Many Men Experience

If you live long enough, your prostate will change.

That is not a warning. It is a simple, honest fact of life.

By the time men reach their 50s and 60s, a large number of them have some degree of prostate enlargement. Some notice symptoms early. Others may remain comfortable for years.

This condition is called **benign prostatic hyperplasia**, or BPH.

Let me say this clearly at the beginning.

BPH is not cancer. It does not turn into cancer.

Understanding this removes a large part of the fear that many men carry.

What Does Enlargement Really Mean?

The prostate surrounds the urethra, the channel through which urine flows.

As the prostate enlarges, it presses inward on this channel.

Even a modest increase in size can create noticeable changes in urine flow.

So the issue is not just how big the prostate becomes.

It is how that growth affects the passage of urine and how the bladder responds.

Why Does the Prostate Grow?

The exact cause is not fully understood, but hormones play an important role.

As men age, the balance of testosterone and related hormones changes. This leads to gradual growth of prostate tissue.

This process is slow and natural.

Not every man develops symptoms, but many do.

How BPH Leads to Symptoms

As the prostate presses on the urethra:

- Urine flow becomes restricted
- The bladder must push harder
- The bladder becomes more sensitive

This leads to a combination of symptoms:

- Weak or slow stream
- Difficulty starting urination
- Frequent urination
- Urgency
- Night-time urination
- Feeling of incomplete emptying

Over time, the bladder itself may change, adding to these symptoms.

Why Size and Symptoms Do Not Always Match

This is an important point that often surprises people.

A man with a large prostate may have mild symptoms.
A man with a smaller prostate may have severe symptoms.

Why?

Because symptoms depend on:

- The degree of obstruction
- The behavior of the bladder
- Individual sensitivity

So treatment decisions are based on symptoms and impact on life, not size alone.

Mild, Moderate, and Severe Symptoms

Doctors often classify symptoms into three levels.

Mild
Symptoms are present but do not significantly affect daily life.

Moderate
Symptoms begin to disturb sleep, comfort, or routine.

Severe
Symptoms interfere with daily activities or lead to complications.

This helps guide the choice of treatment.

When Observation Is Enough

Not every case needs immediate treatment.

If symptoms are mild, a simple approach may be enough:

- Monitor symptoms
- Make lifestyle adjustments
- Have regular follow-up

Many men remain stable for long periods with this approach.

When Treatment Becomes Necessary

Treatment is considered when:

- Symptoms disturb sleep or daily life
- Urination becomes difficult
- There is incomplete bladder emptying
- Complications begin to develop

The goal is to improve comfort and prevent long-term problems.

Common Everyday Factors That Worsen Symptoms

Many men unknowingly make their symptoms worse.

These include:

- Drinking large amounts of fluid late in the evening
- Excess caffeine or alcohol
- Constipation
- Delaying medical care

Simple changes can bring noticeable improvement.

A Reflection From Practice

A man in his mid-fifties came with mild symptoms.

He was waking up twice at night and had a slightly weak stream.

Instead of starting medication immediately, we adjusted his evening fluid intake and reduced caffeine.

Within a few weeks, his symptoms improved.

He avoided medication simply by understanding his habits.

Doctor's Pearl

Enlarged prostate is a common part of aging. The key is not to fear it, but to manage it thoughtfully and early.

Chapter Summary

- BPH is a common, non-cancerous enlargement of the prostate
- It is related to aging and hormonal changes
- Symptoms result from pressure on the urethra and bladder response
- Symptom severity does not always match prostate size
- Many cases can be managed with observation and lifestyle changes

- Treatment is needed when symptoms affect quality of life

Action Plan

- Pay attention to how symptoms affect your daily routine
- Do not assume all enlargement is dangerous
- Try simple lifestyle changes if symptoms are mild
- Seek medical advice if symptoms persist or worsen
- Take a balanced and proactive approach

Now that you understand enlarged prostate clearly, the next step is to focus on what you can do yourself.

In the next chapter, we will discuss practical lifestyle changes that can improve symptoms and support long-term prostate health.

CHAPTER 11: Lifestyle Changes That Truly Help – Simple Steps With Real Impact

Where Real Improvement Often Begins

When men think about treatment, they often think about medicines or procedures.

But in my experience, some of the most meaningful improvements begin much earlier, with simple changes in daily habits.

These are not complicated. They do not require special equipment. But when done consistently, they can reduce symptoms, improve comfort, and sometimes delay the need for medication.

This chapter is about those practical, realistic steps.

Fluid Timing: A Small Change With Big Results

Most people focus on how much water they drink.

But timing matters just as much.

If you drink large amounts of fluid in the evening, especially close to bedtime, you are likely to wake up at night to urinate.

A simple adjustment can help:

- Drink most fluids earlier in the day
- Reduce intake 2 to 3 hours before sleep

This one step alone can reduce night-time urination for many men.

Caffeine and Alcohol: Common Triggers

Caffeine and alcohol can irritate the bladder and increase urinary symptoms.

They may lead to:

- Increased urgency
- More frequent urination
- Night-time awakenings

Common sources include:

- Coffee
- Tea
- Soft drinks
- Alcoholic beverages

You do not need to stop completely, but moderation is important, especially in the evening.

LIFESTYLE CHANGES FOR PROSTATE HEALTH

Simple daily habits can improve symptoms and support a healthy prostate.

1. MANAGE FLUIDS

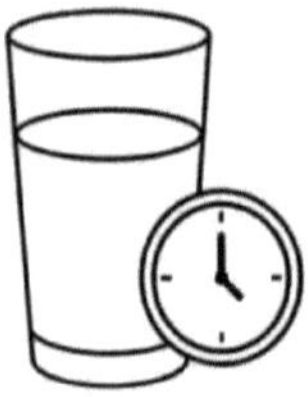

- Drink enough water daily.
- Avoid excess fluids in the evening.
- Limit caffeine and alcohol.

2. STAY ACTIVE

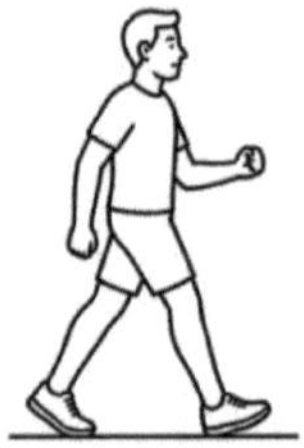

- Exercise regularly.
- Helps improve urine flow and overall health.
- Aim for at least 30 minutes a day.

3. EAT A HEALTHY DIET

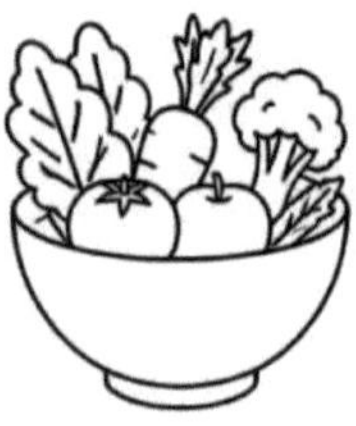

- Eat more fruits, vegetables and whole grains.
- Choose healthy fats (olive oil, nuts, seeds).
- Limit red meat and processed foods.

4. MAINTAIN A HEALTHY WEIGHT

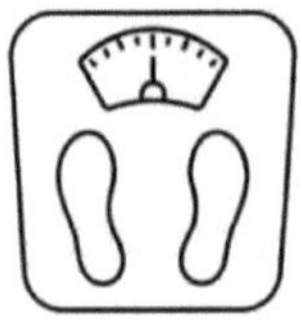

- Excess weight can worsen symptoms.
- Healthy weight supports better hormone balance and prostate health.

5. GET GOOD SLEEP

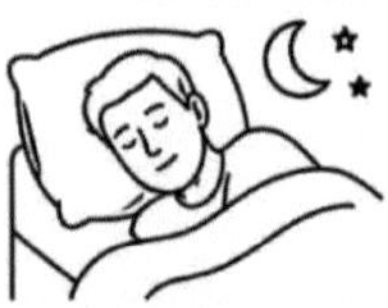

- Poor sleep can worsen symptoms.
- Aim for 7–8 hours of quality sleep.
- Reduce screen time before bed.

6. REDUCE STRESS

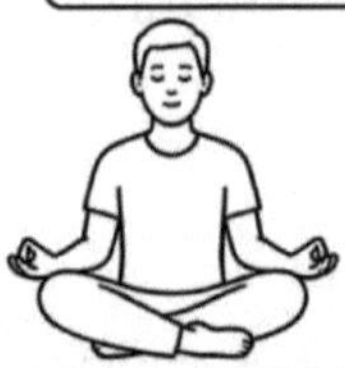

- Stress can worsen urinary symptoms.
- Practice relaxation techniques.
- Yoga, meditation and deep breathing can help.

KEY TAKEAWAY

Healthy lifestyle habits can reduce symptoms, improve quality of life and support long-term prostate health.

Weight and Physical Activity: Quiet but Powerful Factors

Excess weight increases pressure on the abdomen and bladder.

It is also associated with more severe urinary symptoms.

Regular physical activity helps:

- Improve bladder function
- Support overall metabolic health
- Improve sleep
- Reduce stress

You do not need an intense program.

A daily walk or light exercise is enough to begin seeing benefits.

Constipation: Often Overlooked

Many men do not realize that bowel habits affect urinary symptoms.

Constipation increases pressure in the pelvic region, which can worsen urinary problems.

Simple steps include:

- Increasing fiber intake
- Maintaining regular bowel habits
- Staying hydrated during the day

Improving bowel health often improves urinary comfort.

Sleep Routine: Supporting Recovery

Sleep and prostate symptoms are closely connected.

Poor sleep makes symptoms feel worse, and symptoms disturb sleep.

You can improve this cycle by:

- Keeping a regular sleep schedule
- Avoiding heavy meals before bedtime
- Limiting screen time at night

Better sleep improves overall well-being.

Stress and the Body

Stress affects the body in subtle but important ways.

It can increase muscle tension, including in the pelvic region, and make urgency or discomfort feel worse.

Managing stress may include:

- Regular physical activity
- Relaxation techniques
- Taking breaks during the day

Reducing stress helps the body respond better.

Bladder Training: Regaining Control

In some men, the bladder becomes overly sensitive.

Bladder training can help improve control.

This involves:

- Gradually increasing the time between urination
- Avoiding the habit of going "just in case"
- Allowing the bladder to hold urine for longer periods

This takes patience but can be effective.

Common Mistakes to Avoid

Many men unintentionally worsen their symptoms.

Avoid these habits:

- Drinking excessive fluids late in the evening
- Consuming high amounts of caffeine
- Ignoring constipation
- Delaying medical evaluation
- Taking medications without guidance

Awareness is the first step toward improvement.

A Reflection From Practice

A patient in his early sixties came with frequent urination and poor sleep.

He was drinking multiple cups of tea in the evening and large amounts of water before bedtime.

We made simple adjustments.

Within a few weeks, his symptoms improved significantly.

He did not need medication.

Doctor's Pearl

Simple lifestyle changes may seem small, but when practiced consistently, they can have a powerful effect on symptoms and quality of life.

Chapter Summary

- Fluid timing plays an important role in night-time urination
- Caffeine and alcohol can worsen symptoms
- Healthy weight and activity improve urinary function
- Constipation can aggravate symptoms
- Sleep and stress influence overall well-being
- Bladder training can improve control

Action Plan

- Shift most fluid intake to earlier in the day
- Reduce caffeine and alcohol, especially in the evening
- Stay physically active with simple daily exercise
- Maintain regular bowel habits
- Improve sleep routine
- Manage stress
- Avoid habits that worsen symptoms

Now that you understand how lifestyle changes can help, the next step is to explore medical treatment options.

In the next chapter, we will discuss medications for enlarged prostate, how they work, and what you can expect from them.

CHAPTER 12: Medications for Enlarged Prostate – What Works, What to Expect

When Lifestyle Changes Are Not Enough

Many men do quite well with simple lifestyle adjustments.

But sometimes, despite doing everything right, symptoms continue to disturb sleep, daily comfort, and overall quality of life.

This is when medications become helpful.

Let me set the right expectation from the beginning.

Medications do not "cure" prostate enlargement. They control symptoms and improve comfort.

For many men, that is exactly what is needed.

The Two Main Types of Medications

Most treatments for an enlarged prostate fall into two main groups:

- Alpha blockers
- 5-alpha reductase inhibitors

Sometimes one is used. Sometimes both are combined.

Once you understand these two, everything else becomes easier.

Alpha Blockers: Quick Relief for Urine Flow

These are often the first medicines prescribed.

They work by relaxing the muscles around the prostate and the bladder outlet. When these muscles relax, urine can flow more freely.

What you may notice:

- Improved urine stream
- Less difficulty starting urination
- Reduced urgency

These medicines act relatively quickly. Many men feel improvement within a few days to a couple of weeks.

Possible side effects:

- Lightheadedness, especially when standing up quickly
- Tiredness
- Changes in ejaculation in some men

Most side effects are mild and can be managed.

5-Alpha Reductase Inhibitors: Working on the Size

These medicines work in a different way.

They gradually shrink the prostate by reducing the effect of certain hormones.

What to expect:

- Slower onset of action
- Improvement over several months
- Reduced risk of progression over time

These are particularly useful in men with larger prostates.

Possible side effects:

- Reduced sexual desire in some men
- Erectile difficulty in a minority
- Reduced semen volume

Not everyone experiences these effects, but it is important to be aware.

Combination Therapy: Using Both Approaches

In some cases, both types of medicines are used together.

This approach offers:

- Faster symptom relief from alpha blockers
- Long-term benefit from size reduction

It is often recommended when symptoms are more significant or when the prostate is clearly enlarged.

Medications for Bladder Symptoms

Sometimes symptoms are driven more by bladder behavior than by obstruction.

In such cases, additional medicines may be used to calm an overactive bladder.

This is why treatment is personalized.

Not every patient receives the same combination.

How to Know If Treatment Is Working

Improvement is not measured only by tests.

It shows in daily life:

- Better sleep
- Fewer trips to the bathroom
- Improved comfort while urinating
- Less urgency

Some men expect immediate results. It is better to expect gradual, steady improvement.

When Medications Are Not Enough

Medications work well for many men, but not for all.

If symptoms remain troublesome or complications develop, procedures may be needed.

This does not mean failure.

It simply means the condition requires a different approach.

A Reflection From Practice

A 66-year-old patient came with moderate symptoms and poor sleep.

We started an alpha blocker.

Within two weeks, his night-time urination reduced, and he began sleeping better.

Later, we added a second medication to address prostate size.

He remained comfortable and avoided surgery.

Doctor's Pearl

Medications are not about perfection. They are about meaningful improvement in daily life.

Chapter Summary

- Medications are used when lifestyle changes are not enough
- Alpha blockers provide quick relief
- 5-alpha reductase inhibitors reduce prostate size over time
- Combination therapy may offer added benefit
- Side effects are usually mild and manageable
- Treatment is tailored to the individual

Action Plan

- Discuss medication options openly with your doctor
- Understand both benefits and possible side effects
- Give treatment enough time to work
- Report any bothersome side effects
- Continue lifestyle measures along with medication

Now that you understand medications, the next step is to explore what happens when symptoms persist despite treatment.

In the next chapter, we will discuss procedures and surgical options in a clear and reassuring way.

CHAPTER 13: Procedures and Surgery – When Relief Needs a Stronger Step

Moving Beyond Medicines, Without Fear

For many men, medications bring steady relief.

But sometimes, symptoms continue to disturb sleep, daily comfort, and confidence. In other cases, complications begin to appear.

This is when we consider procedures or surgery.

Let me reassure you at the beginning.

These treatments are common, effective, and much less intimidating than most people imagine.

The goal is simple. Restore comfortable urine flow and improve quality of life.

When a Procedure Becomes Necessary

Your doctor may suggest a procedure if:

- Symptoms remain moderate to severe despite medication
- Side effects of medicines are difficult to tolerate

- You develop urinary retention
- Infections occur repeatedly
- The bladder is not emptying well
- Daily life is clearly affected

The decision is not rushed. It is based on how much the condition is affecting you.

The Core Principle Behind All Procedures

All procedures aim to solve the same problem.

They create more space for urine to pass.

This can be done by:

- Removing excess prostate tissue
- Vaporizing or shrinking tissue
- Repositioning tissue to open the urinary channel

Once the blockage is relieved, the bladder no longer needs to struggle.

TURP: A Time-Tested Standard

TURP stands for transurethral resection of the prostate.

It has been used for many years and remains one of the most reliable treatments.

What happens:

- A thin instrument is passed through the urethra
- Excess prostate tissue is carefully removed
- No external cuts are required

What you can expect:

- Strong improvement in urine flow
- Significant symptom relief
- Durable results over time

Possible side effects:

- Temporary burning during urination
- Retrograde ejaculation
- Rare bleeding or infection

For many men, this procedure restores comfort and normal routine.

Laser Treatments: Modern and Effective

Laser procedures use focused energy to remove or vaporize prostate tissue.

Advantages include:

- Less bleeding
- Shorter hospital stay
- Faster recovery

In many cases, results are similar to TURP.

These procedures have become increasingly popular.

TREATMENT OPTIONS FOR PROSTATE PROBLEMS

Treatment depends on the cause, severity of symptoms, age, and overall health.

1 LIFESTYLE CHANGES

- Healthy diet
- Regular exercise
- Weight management
- Limit caffeine and alcohol
- Good sleep and stress control

2 MEDICATIONS

- Alpha blockers – relax muscles, improve urine flow
- 5-Alpha reductase inhibitors – shrink prostate over time
- Other medications for specific symptoms

3 MINIMALLY INVASIVE PROCEDURES

- UroLift
- Rezūm (water vapor therapy)
- Prostatic artery embolization (PAE)
- Shorter recovery time

4 SURGICAL OPTIONS

- TURP (Transurethral Resection of the Prostate)
- Laser surgery
- Open or robotic prostatectomy (mainly for prostate cancer)

5 ACTIVE SURVEILLANCE

- For low-risk prostate cancer
- Regular PSA tests, exams and imaging
- Treatment started only if needed

6 SUPPORTIVE CARE

- Manage symptoms
- Improve quality of life
- Ongoing follow-up and support

IMPORTANT POINTS

Consult your doctor to choose the right option for you.

Goal is to relieve symptoms, prevent complications and improve quality of life.

Early treatment can prevent problems from getting worse.

Regular follow-up is important for long-term health.

KEY TAKEAWAY

Many effective treatment options are available.
Work with your doctor to find the best plan for your health, needs and goals.

Minimally Invasive Options

Newer techniques aim to provide relief with minimal disruption.

These may include:

- Methods that gently move prostate tissue away from the urethra
- Techniques that use heat or steam to shrink tissue

Advantages:

- Often done as outpatient procedures
- Faster return to daily activities
- Lower risk of certain side effects

However, not every patient is a candidate. The choice depends on prostate size, symptoms, and overall health.

What Recovery Feels Like

Recovery depends on the type of procedure.

In the early phase, you may notice:

- Mild burning during urination
- Increased frequency
- Gradual improvement over weeks

Most men begin to feel significant relief within a few weeks.

Patience during this period is important.

Understanding Risks in Perspective

Every procedure carries some risk.

But serious complications are uncommon.

Possible concerns include:

- Temporary urinary symptoms during healing
- Changes in ejaculation
- Rare infection or bleeding

The key is proper patient selection and experienced care.

A Reflection From Practice

A man in his late sixties had severe symptoms.

He was waking up four to five times each night and had difficulty emptying his bladder.

He had delayed treatment for years.

After a minimally invasive procedure, his symptoms improved significantly. He began sleeping through the night again.

His only regret was waiting too long.

Doctor's Pearl

A well-timed procedure can restore comfort, improve sleep, and greatly enhance quality of life. Do not see it as a failure, but as the right next step when needed.

Chapter Summary

- Procedures are considered when medicines are not enough
- The goal is to relieve obstruction and improve urine flow
- TURP is a reliable and effective option
- Laser procedures offer similar benefits with faster recovery
- Minimally invasive options are available for selected patients
- Most men experience significant improvement

Action Plan

- Do not fear procedures if symptoms are affecting your life
- Discuss all available options with your doctor
- Understand benefits, risks, and recovery expectations
- Choose the option that fits your needs
- Seek timely care rather than delaying

Now that you understand treatment for an enlarged prostate, we move to another important condition.

In the next chapter, we will discuss prostatitis, a condition that often causes pain and discomfort and is frequently misunderstood.

CHAPTER 14: Prostatitis and Chronic Pelvic Pain – Understanding the Unpredictable

A Condition That Does Not Follow Rules

By now, you have seen that enlarged prostate and cancer follow clearer patterns.

Prostatitis is different.

It does not always behave in a predictable way. Symptoms may appear, improve, return, and sometimes change in intensity. Tests may be normal, yet the discomfort is very real.

This uncertainty is what makes prostatitis frustrating.

But there is something reassuring you must understand.

Most forms of prostatitis are not dangerous. They are uncomfortable, sometimes persistent, but manageable.

What Prostatitis Really Means

The word may sound complex, but the meaning is simple.

Prostatitis means **inflammation of the prostate**.

The challenge is that this inflammation can occur for different reasons, and not all of them involve infection.

That is why prostatitis is not one single disease. It is a group of related conditions.

The Main Types, Made Simple

You do not need to remember technical terms, but understanding the basic types helps.

Acute bacterial prostatitis
This is caused by infection and comes on suddenly.

Symptoms may include:

- Fever and chills
- Burning urination
- Pelvic pain
- Difficulty passing urine

This condition needs prompt treatment.

Chronic bacterial prostatitis
Here, infection persists or recurs.

Symptoms are usually milder but repeated:

- Recurrent urinary discomfort

- Episodes of infection
- Ongoing irritation

Chronic pelvic pain syndrome (most common)
This is the most confusing form.

You may have:

- Persistent pelvic discomfort
- Urinary symptoms
- Pain during or after ejaculation

But tests may not show infection.

This does not mean nothing is wrong. It means the problem is more complex.

Common Symptoms You May Notice

Prostatitis often presents with discomfort.

Typical symptoms include:

- Burning or pain during urination
- Pain in the lower abdomen, pelvis, or back
- Discomfort in the groin or perineal area
- Pain during or after ejaculation
- Frequent or urgent urination

Unlike enlarged prostate, **pain is a key feature**.

Why It Feels So Confusing

Many men expect a clear answer.

"Is it infection or not?"

But prostatitis does not always fit that pattern.

- Tests may be normal
- Antibiotics may not always help
- Symptoms may fluctuate

This can be frustrating, but it is part of the nature of this condition.

What Causes Ongoing Symptoms

In many cases, there is not a single cause.

It may involve a combination of:

- Past infection
- Muscle tension in the pelvic floor
- Nerve sensitivity
- Stress and emotional factors

It is best understood as a condition involving both body and function.

How Diagnosis Is Made

Diagnosis focuses on:

- Understanding symptoms carefully
- Examining the prostate
- Checking urine for infection

Additional tests may be done to rule out other conditions.

The goal is not only to find infection, but to understand the pattern.

Treatment: Why Patience Is Important

Treatment depends on the type.

For bacterial prostatitis:

- Antibiotics are required

For chronic pelvic pain syndrome:

- Treatment is individualized
- May include medications, relaxation techniques, and lifestyle changes

Improvement is often gradual.

Understanding this prevents frustration.

Simple Measures That Help

Many men benefit from practical steps:

- Warm baths to relax muscles
- Avoiding prolonged sitting
- Gentle physical activity
- Managing stress

These may seem simple, but they can significantly reduce symptoms.

The Mind-Body Connection

Stress can increase muscle tension in the pelvic area.

This can worsen symptoms.

Addressing stress does not mean the problem is "in the mind."

It means the body and mind are connected.

Managing stress can reduce physical discomfort.

A Reflection From Practice

A man in his forties came with persistent pelvic discomfort.

He had taken multiple courses of antibiotics without relief.

After careful evaluation, we focused on relaxation, lifestyle changes, and stress control.

Gradually, his symptoms improved.

The key was understanding the condition rather than repeating the same treatment.

Doctor's Pearl

Prostatitis often requires patience and a broader approach. Quick fixes are uncommon, but steady improvement is achievable.

Chapter Summary

- Prostatitis means inflammation of the prostate
- It includes acute infection, chronic infection, and chronic pain syndromes
- Pain is a key feature
- Diagnosis is based on symptoms and basic tests
- Treatment depends on the type
- Chronic forms require patience and a holistic approach

Action Plan

- Do not panic if symptoms persist but tests are normal
- Seek proper evaluation rather than repeated self-treatment
- Follow treatment plans consistently
- Pay attention to stress and lifestyle factors
- Be patient, as improvement takes time

Now that you understand prostatitis, we will move to the condition that creates the most concern.

In the next chapter, we will discuss prostate cancer in a clear and balanced way, so that you can understand it without unnecessary fear.

CHAPTER 15: Prostate Cancer – Clear Understanding Without Fear

The Word That Creates Immediate Anxiety

The moment the word "cancer" is mentioned, the mind reacts.

Worry comes quickly. Questions follow. Many men begin to imagine the worst.

I have seen this reaction countless times in my practice.

But when it comes to prostate cancer, the reality is more balanced than most people expect.

Let me begin with a simple truth.

Not all prostate cancers behave the same way.

This one idea changes everything.

How Common Is Prostate Cancer?

Prostate cancer is one of the most common cancers in men, especially after the age of 50.

But there is another important fact.

Many men who are diagnosed with prostate cancer live long, healthy lives, particularly when the disease is detected early and behaves in a slow, controlled manner.

So while the diagnosis is important, it is not always urgent.

Why Prostate Cancer Is Different From Many Others

Unlike many cancers, prostate cancer has a wide range of behavior.

Some cancers:

- Grow very slowly
- Remain confined to the prostate
- May never cause harm

Others:

- Grow more quickly
- Spread beyond the prostate
- Require active treatment

This variation is the reason careful evaluation is essential before making decisions.

Risk Factors You Should Know

Certain factors increase the likelihood of prostate cancer:

- Increasing age
- Family history of prostate cancer
- Genetic influences
- Certain racial backgrounds

Among these, age is the most important.

Risk increases steadily as men grow older.

Symptoms: Often Silent in Early Stages

One of the most important points to understand is this:

Early prostate cancer usually does not cause symptoms.

That is why it is often detected through PSA testing or routine evaluation.

When symptoms do appear, they may include:

- Difficulty with urination
- Blood in urine
- Bone pain in advanced stages

These are usually later findings.

How Prostate Cancer Is Diagnosed

Diagnosis involves several steps:

- PSA blood test
- Physical examination
- Imaging, such as MRI
- Biopsy for confirmation

No single test gives the full answer.

It is the combination that provides clarity.

Understanding Grade and Stage

After diagnosis, doctors assess two key aspects.

Grade
This reflects how aggressive the cancer cells appear under the microscope.

Higher grade means more aggressive behavior.

Stage
This describes how far the cancer has spread.

If it is confined to the prostate, it is localized. If it spreads beyond, it is more advanced.

These two factors guide treatment decisions.

Why Some Cancers Do Not Need Immediate Treatment

This is one of the most important ideas in prostate care.

Some prostate cancers grow so slowly that immediate treatment is not necessary.

In such cases, doctors may recommend **active surveillance**.

This involves:

- Regular monitoring
- PSA testing
- Periodic imaging or biopsy

The goal is to avoid unnecessary treatment while keeping the situation under control.

The Emotional Side of Diagnosis

Even when the cancer is low-risk, the emotional impact can be strong.

You may feel:

- Fear
- Anxiety
- Uncertainty

These reactions are natural.

But understanding the nature of the disease helps reduce unnecessary worry and allows for clearer thinking.

PROSTATE CANCER

Understand. Detect Early. Treat Effectively.

WHAT IS IT?

Prostate cancer begins in the prostate gland. It often grows slowly and may not cause problems early on.

RISK FACTORS

- Age over 50
- Family history
- Genetics
- African American race

SYMPTOMS

- Frequent urination
- Weak or slow urine flow
- Difficulty starting or stopping urine
- Blood in urine or semen
- Pain in back, hips or pelvis

SCREENING

- PSA blood test
- Digital Rectal Examination (DRE)
- Talk to your doctor about when to start screening

TREATMENT OPTIONS

ACTIVE SURVEILLANCE

- For low-risk, slow-growing cancer
- Regular PSA tests, exams and imaging
- Treatment started only if needed

SURGERY

- Remove the prostate gland
- Robotic-assisted or open prostatectomy
- Effective for localized cancer

RADIATION THERAPY

- Destroys cancer cells with high-energy rays
- External beam radiation or brachytherapy
- Effective for localized cancer

HORMONE THERAPY

- Lowers levels of male hormones (androgens)
- Slows cancer growth
- Used for advanced or recurrent cancer

OTHER TREATMENTS

- Chemotherapy
- Immunotherapy
- Targeted therapy
- Used in advanced or metastatic cancer

IMPORTANT POINTS

- Early detection increases the chance of successful treatment.
- Many prostate cancers grow slowly and may not need immediate treatment.
- Discuss risks, benefits and side effects with your doctor.
- Healthy lifestyle supports overall well-being during treatment.
- Regular follow-up is important for monitoring and adjusting care.

KEY TAKEAWAY

Prostate cancer is treatable, especially when detected early.
Work with your healthcare team to choose the best plan for you.

A Reflection From Practice

A man in his early sixties was diagnosed with low-risk prostate cancer.

He expected immediate surgery.

After discussion, he chose active surveillance.

Years later, his condition remained stable, and he avoided treatment-related side effects.

This is not uncommon.

Doctor's Pearl

A diagnosis of prostate cancer is not always a race against time. It is a condition that requires careful understanding and thoughtful decision-making.

Chapter Summary

- Prostate cancer is common, especially with age
- Not all prostate cancers are aggressive
- Early stages often have no symptoms
- Diagnosis involves PSA, examination, imaging, and biopsy
- Grade and stage determine severity
- Some cancers can be safely monitored without immediate treatment

Action Plan

- Do not panic if prostate cancer is suspected or diagnosed
- Focus on understanding the nature of the cancer
- Discuss all options, including observation
- Seek clear and reliable information
- Make decisions based on understanding, not fear

Now that you understand prostate cancer clearly, the next step is to explore how it is treated.

In the next chapter, we will discuss treatment options in a simple and practical way, so you can understand what each option means and how to choose wisely.

CHAPTER 16: Prostate Cancer Treatment – Choosing the Right Path for You

There Is No Single "Best" Treatment

When men hear they have cancer, the natural instinct is to act quickly.

"Remove it."
"Treat it immediately."

That reaction is understandable.

But prostate cancer is different from many other conditions.

The best treatment is not the most aggressive one. It is the one that fits your specific cancer and your life.

Taking time to understand your options often leads to better outcomes and greater peace of mind.

How Treatment Decisions Are Made

Before choosing treatment, several important factors are considered:

- How aggressive the cancer is
- Whether it is confined to the prostate or has spread
- PSA levels and their trend
- Your age and overall health
- Your personal priorities and preferences

Treatment is not chosen in isolation. It is tailored to you.

Active Surveillance: Careful Monitoring

For many men with low-risk cancer, immediate treatment is not necessary.

Active surveillance means:

- Regular PSA testing
- Periodic imaging
- Occasional biopsy if needed

The goal is to monitor the cancer and treat only if it shows signs of progression.

Benefits:

- Avoids unnecessary side effects
- Maintains quality of life

This is a thoughtful and safe option for many men.

Surgery: Removing the Prostate

Surgery, known as prostatectomy, involves removing the prostate gland.

It is usually considered when:

- Cancer is localized
- The patient prefers a definitive approach
- Overall health supports surgery

Benefits:

- Removes the cancer if confined
- Provides detailed information about the disease

Possible side effects:

- Urinary leakage
- Erectile dysfunction

These effects vary and often improve over time.

Radiation Therapy: Treating Without Surgery

Radiation therapy uses high-energy rays to destroy cancer cells.

It may be delivered as:

- External beam radiation
- Internal radiation, known as brachytherapy

Benefits:

- No major surgery
- Effective for many stages of cancer

Possible side effects:

- Urinary irritation
- Bowel changes
- Gradual impact on sexual function

Radiation is a strong alternative to surgery.

Hormone Therapy: Slowing Cancer Growth

Prostate cancer often depends on male hormones for growth.

Hormone therapy reduces or blocks these hormones.

It is used:

- In more advanced cancer
- Along with radiation in certain cases

Possible effects:

- Fatigue
- Reduced sexual desire
- Changes in body composition

It is usually part of a broader treatment plan.

Treatment for Advanced Disease

When cancer has spread beyond the prostate, treatment focuses on:

- Slowing progression
- Controlling symptoms
- Maintaining quality of life

Options may include:

- Hormone therapy
- Chemotherapy
- Newer targeted treatments

These treatments have improved significantly in recent years.

Balancing Benefits and Side Effects

Every treatment offers benefits and carries potential risks.

The decision often involves balancing:

- Effectiveness of treatment
- Impact on urinary function
- Impact on sexual health
- Overall quality of life

There is no perfect answer.

There is a **personal answer**.

What Matters Most to Patients

In real life, patients often care deeply about:

- Living longer
- Maintaining independence
- Preserving bladder control
- Preserving sexual function

These concerns are valid and should guide decisions.

A Reflection From Practice

Two patients with similar diagnoses chose different paths.

One chose surgery for a clear, single-step approach.
The other chose radiation to avoid an operation.

Both understood their options.

Both were satisfied with their decisions.

That is what matters.

Doctor's Pearl

Do not rush into treatment out of fear. A thoughtful decision, based on understanding, often leads to better outcomes.

Chapter Summary

- Treatment depends on cancer type, stage, and patient factors
- Active surveillance is appropriate for many low-risk cases
- Surgery removes the prostate and may cure localized cancer
- Radiation is an effective alternative to surgery
- Hormone therapy is used in advanced or combined treatment
- Decisions should balance benefits and side effects

Action Plan

- Take time to understand your diagnosis
- Discuss all treatment options clearly
- Consider your lifestyle and priorities
- Ask questions until you are comfortable
- Choose a treatment path with confidence

Now that you understand treatment options, the next step is to look at life after treatment.

In the next chapter, we will discuss how prostate conditions and their treatments affect urination, sexual health, and overall quality of life, and how these can be managed effectively.

CHAPTER 17: Life After Treatment – Regaining Control and Confidence

What Most Men Quietly Worry About

After the discussion of treatment, a different set of questions begins to surface.

They are not always spoken openly, but they are deeply felt.

"Will I be able to control my urine?"
"What will happen to my sexual life?"
"Will I feel like myself again?"

These are not small concerns. They affect daily life, relationships, and self-confidence.

Let us talk about them clearly and honestly.

Urinary Control: What to Expect

After certain treatments, especially surgery, it is common to have some difficulty controlling urine in the early phase.

You may notice:

- Leakage during coughing, laughing, or movement

- Need for protective pads
- Occasional urgency

This can feel discouraging.

But in most cases, this is temporary.

With time and proper exercises, control improves steadily over weeks to months.

Pelvic Floor Exercises: A Key Part of Recovery

One of the most effective ways to regain control is strengthening the pelvic floor muscles.

These muscles help regulate urination.

Regular pelvic floor exercises can:

- Improve bladder control
- Speed recovery
- Increase confidence

The key is consistency.

Even a few minutes daily can make a meaningful difference.

Changes in Urination Pattern

After treatment, especially procedures that relieve blockage, many men notice:

- A stronger urine stream
- Better emptying of the bladder

During early recovery, you may also experience:

- Mild burning
- Increased frequency

These usually improve as healing progresses.

Sexual Health: Understanding the Changes

Sexual function is an important part of overall well-being.

The impact of treatment varies depending on:

- Type of treatment
- Age
- Overall health

Each person's experience is different.

Erectile Function

Erections depend on delicate nerves near the prostate.

These nerves may be affected during treatment.

You may experience:

- Temporary difficulty with erections
- Gradual improvement over time
- In some cases, longer-term changes

Supportive treatments are available, and many men improve with time.

Changes in Ejaculation

After certain treatments:

- Ejaculation may change
- Semen release may be reduced or absent

This does not eliminate the ability to feel pleasure, but it is important to understand in advance.

Emotional and Relationship Impact

Physical changes often affect emotional well-being.

You may feel:

- Reduced confidence
- Concern about intimacy
- Hesitation in relationships

Open communication with your partner is important.

Understanding and support make adjustment easier.

Recovery Takes Time

Many men expect a quick return to normal.

In reality, recovery is gradual.

There may be good days and less comfortable days.

What matters is the overall direction, which is usually toward improvement.

Patience is essential.

Support Systems Matter

You do not have to manage this alone.

Support may come from:

- Your doctor
- Your partner
- Counseling when needed

With proper support, most men adapt well and regain confidence.

A Reflection From Practice

A patient in his mid-sixties was very concerned about urinary leakage after surgery.

In the early weeks, he needed pads and felt frustrated.

With time and regular exercises, his control improved significantly.

Later, he said his biggest mistake was worrying too much in the beginning.

Doctor's Pearl

Recovery is a process, not an event. Patience and consistency are as important as treatment itself.

Chapter Summary

- Urinary leakage may occur after treatment but often improves
- Pelvic floor exercises help restore control
- Sexual function may be affected but can improve
- Ejaculation changes are common
- Emotional well-being and relationships are important
- Recovery takes time and patience

Action Plan

- Begin pelvic floor exercises as advised
- Be patient with your recovery
- Discuss sexual concerns openly with your doctor
- Communicate with your partner
- Focus on gradual improvement

You have now understood the major conditions and treatments related to prostate health.

In the next chapter, we will shift the focus to prevention and healthy aging, so you can take practical steps to protect your prostate and overall health in the years ahead.

CHAPTER 18: Prevention and Healthy Aging – Taking Charge of Your Prostate Health

A Question Almost Every Man Asks

"Doctor, how can I prevent prostate problems?"

It is a thoughtful question, and it comes from a natural desire to stay healthy and avoid disease.

The honest answer is balanced.

You cannot completely prevent all prostate conditions. Aging and genetics play a role that we cannot fully control.

But this is equally important.

You can influence how your prostate behaves, how severe your symptoms become, and how well you age.

That is where your power lies.

Think of the Whole Body, Not Just One Organ

The prostate does not exist in isolation.

Your overall health strongly influences how your body functions, including your prostate.

So instead of focusing only on the prostate, it is more useful to think about:

- Your diet
- Your weight
- Your activity level
- Your sleep
- Your stress

A healthier body supports a healthier prostate.

Diet: Practical, Not Complicated

There is no single food that can prevent prostate disease.

But a balanced pattern of eating supports long-term health.

This includes:

- Plenty of vegetables and fruits
- Whole grains
- Healthy fats such as those from fish and nuts
- Limiting processed and high-fat foods

These habits help reduce inflammation and support overall well-being.

Be cautious of claims that promise quick results.

No single food or supplement can guarantee prevention.

Weight: A Silent Contributor

Excess weight affects many systems in the body.

It increases pressure on the abdomen and bladder and is associated with more severe urinary symptoms.

Maintaining a healthy weight can:

- Reduce urinary symptoms
- Improve energy levels
- Support heart and metabolic health

Even small changes in weight can have a positive impact.

Physical Activity: One of the Best Tools You Have

Regular physical activity is simple but powerful.

It helps:

- Improve bladder function
- Support hormonal balance
- Reduce stress
- Improve sleep

You do not need an intense routine.

A daily walk or consistent light exercise is enough to begin.

The key is regularity.

Smoking and Alcohol: Understanding Their Effects

Smoking affects overall health and blood circulation.

Alcohol can irritate the bladder and worsen urinary symptoms.

Reducing or avoiding these can improve both general and prostate health.

Sleep: Often Ignored, Always Important

Good sleep supports every system in the body.

Poor sleep can:

- Reduce energy
- Affect concentration
- Worsen how symptoms are perceived

Simple steps include:

- Keeping a regular sleep schedule
- Avoiding heavy meals before bedtime
- Limiting screen time at night

Better sleep improves overall well-being.

Stress: The Invisible Factor

Stress influences the body in subtle ways.

It can increase muscle tension, including in the pelvic region, and make symptoms feel worse.

Managing stress may involve:

- Regular activity
- Relaxation techniques
- Taking time to rest

Reducing stress helps your body function more smoothly.

Supplements: A Balanced View

Many supplements are marketed for prostate health.

Some may offer mild symptom relief.

But the scientific evidence is often limited.

Supplements should not replace proper medical care.

Always discuss them with your doctor.

Regular Checkups: Your Safety Net

Prevention is not only about lifestyle.

Regular follow-up is important.

This may include:

- Monitoring symptoms
- Periodic PSA testing when appropriate
- Early evaluation of any changes

Early awareness leads to better outcomes.

Healthy Aging: A Positive Perspective

Aging is natural.

Prostate changes are part of that process.

But aging does not mean losing control of your health.

Many men remain active, productive, and healthy well into later life.

The goal is not perfection.

The goal is awareness, balance, and steady care.

Myth vs Fact

Myth: Diet alone can prevent prostate cancer
Fact: Diet supports health but does not guarantee prevention

Myth: Supplements can replace treatment
Fact: Supplements may help some symptoms but are not a substitute for medical care

Myth: Prostate problems are unavoidable and untreatable
Fact: Most prostate conditions are manageable with proper care

---

A Reflection From Practice

A man in his late fifties came with early urinary symptoms.

He improved his diet, reduced caffeine, lost weight, and started daily walking.

His symptoms improved enough that he did not need medication for years.

Lifestyle does not solve everything, but it often changes the course.

Doctor's Pearl

You may not control aging, but you can influence how you age. Small, consistent habits create lasting health.

Chapter Summary

- Complete prevention is not always possible
- Healthy lifestyle habits improve outcomes
- Diet, weight, and activity play key roles
- Smoking and alcohol can worsen symptoms
- Sleep and stress affect overall well-being
- Supplements should be used cautiously
- Regular checkups support early detection

Action Plan

- Follow a balanced and practical diet
- Maintain a healthy weight
- Stay physically active
- Reduce caffeine, alcohol, and smoking
- Improve sleep habits
- Manage stress
- Schedule regular medical checkups

You have now learned how to support your prostate and overall health.

In the next chapter, we will look ahead at new research and future directions in prostate care, so you understand how medicine is evolving and what that means for you.

CHAPTER 19: New Research and the Future of Prostate Care – What Lies Ahead

Why It Helps to Look Forward

Medicine is always moving.

What we understood ten or twenty years ago has already changed. The tools we use today are more precise, less invasive, and better tailored to individual needs.

The direction is clear.

Prostate care is becoming more accurate, more personalized, and less disruptive.

You do not need to follow every new development. But understanding the direction helps you make better decisions and have more informed conversations with your doctor.

From Standard Care to Personalized Care

In the past, treatment decisions often followed general guidelines.

Today, the focus is shifting toward the individual.

Doctors now ask:

- How aggressive is this specific cancer?
- What is the patient's overall health and preference?
- Can treatment be safely delayed or avoided?

This approach reduces unnecessary treatment and improves quality of life.

Better Imaging: Seeing More Clearly

Imaging has improved significantly.

Modern prostate MRI allows doctors to:

- Identify areas that truly need attention
- Avoid unnecessary biopsies in selected cases
- Target suspicious areas more accurately

This reduces guesswork and improves confidence in diagnosis.

Beyond PSA: Smarter Testing

PSA remains useful, but it is no longer the only tool.

Newer blood and urine tests are being developed to answer a more important question:

Is this cancer likely to behave aggressively?

These tests aim to:

- Reduce unnecessary procedures
- Improve risk assessment
- Guide better decisions

They are still evolving, but they represent meaningful progress.

Genetic Insights: Understanding Risk

We now understand that some prostate cancers are influenced by inherited genetic factors.

In selected patients, genetic testing can:

- Identify higher-risk individuals
- Guide treatment decisions
- Inform family members about their own risk

This is especially useful for men with a strong family history.

Precision Treatment: Treating Less, Preserving More

One promising direction is targeted treatment.

Instead of treating the entire prostate, newer approaches aim to:

- Treat only the affected area
- Preserve surrounding healthy tissue

- Reduce side effects

These techniques are still being refined but offer a more balanced approach.

Advances in Treatment for Advanced Disease

For men with more advanced prostate cancer, treatment options have improved significantly.

Newer therapies include:

- More effective hormone-based treatments
- Targeted therapies
- Selected use of immunotherapy

These advances are helping men live longer with better quality of life.

Less Invasive Options for BPH

Even for non-cancerous enlargement, procedures are becoming simpler.

The trend is toward:

- Shorter hospital stays
- Faster recovery
- Better preservation of normal function

This makes treatment more acceptable and less intimidating.

What This Means for You

All these developments point toward one goal.

Better care with fewer side effects.

But it is important to stay balanced.

Not every new test or treatment is necessary for every patient.

The best care is the right care for your situation.

A Balanced Perspective

New technology adds value, but it does not replace proven methods.

Experienced clinical judgment remains essential.

The best outcomes often come from combining established treatments with carefully selected newer options.

A Reflection From Practice

A patient with a mildly elevated PSA was advised to undergo an MRI before considering biopsy.

The MRI showed no concerning findings.

He avoided an unnecessary procedure and a great deal of anxiety.

This is how modern tools can improve real-life care.

Doctor's Pearl

Progress in medicine is most helpful when it simplifies decisions and reduces unnecessary treatment.

Chapter Summary

- Prostate care is becoming more personalized
- MRI has improved diagnosis and reduced unnecessary procedures
- New tests help refine risk assessment
- Genetic insights guide selected patients
- Targeted treatments aim to reduce side effects
- Advances are improving outcomes even in advanced disease
- A balanced approach remains essential

Action Plan

- Stay informed, but avoid unnecessary worry
- Ask about newer options when appropriate
- Focus on what is relevant to your condition
- Trust a balanced, thoughtful approach
- Make decisions based on understanding

You are now approaching the final step of this journey.

In the next chapter, we will answer common questions and bring everything together into clear, practical guidance for long-term prostate health and peace of mind.

CHAPTER 20: Frequently Asked Questions and Final Guidance – Moving Forward With Confidence

A Calm Closing Conversation

You have now walked through this journey step by step.

You understand the prostate, the common conditions, the tests, the treatments, and the role of lifestyle. But even after all this, a few simple, practical questions often remain.

This final chapter is meant to answer those questions clearly, just as I would in a quiet conversation with a patient.

Common Questions About Symptoms

Is it normal to wake up at night to urinate?
Occasionally, yes. But if it happens regularly, especially more than once or twice, it deserves attention.

Is a weak urine stream always serious?
Not always. It is often due to an enlarged prostate. But if it persists, it should be evaluated.

Can symptoms improve without treatment?
Mild symptoms sometimes improve with lifestyle changes. Persistent symptoms usually need proper guidance.

Common Questions About PSA

If my PSA is high, does it mean cancer?
No. PSA can rise due to many non-cancerous conditions.

How often should I check PSA?
This depends on your age, risk, and previous results. It should be decided with your doctor.

Should I worry about small changes?
Not necessarily. Trends over time are more important than a single value.

Common Questions About Prostate Cancer

Does every prostate cancer need treatment?
No. Some slow-growing cancers can be safely monitored.

Is prostate cancer always life-threatening?
No. Many men live long and healthy lives after diagnosis, especially when detected early.

Can prostate cancer be cured?
In many cases, especially when diagnosed early, treatment can be very effective.

Common Questions About Treatment

Will I definitely need surgery?
No. Many men are managed with observation or medication.

Do all treatments affect sexual function?
Not always. The effect varies depending on the type of treatment and individual factors.

Can I return to a normal life?
In most cases, yes. Recovery may take time, but good quality of life is achievable.

Common Questions About Lifestyle

Can diet alone prevent prostate problems?
No. Diet supports health but cannot completely prevent disease.

Are supplements useful?
Some may help mild symptoms, but evidence is limited. They should not replace proper medical care.

Does exercise help?
Yes. Regular physical activity supports overall and prostate health.

Finding the Right Balance

One of the most important lessons in prostate health is balance.

Too much fear leads to anxiety and rushed decisions. Too little attention leads to delay and missed opportunities.

The right approach lies in between.

Be aware, but not anxious.
Be proactive, but not fearful.

A Practical Way to Move Forward

Prostate health is not a one-time decision.

It is a long-term process that includes:

- Paying attention to symptoms
- Having regular medical checkups
- Making thoughtful lifestyle choices
- Acting when needed

This steady approach works better than reacting only when problems become severe.

A Reflection From Years of Practice

Over the years, I have seen two extremes.

Some men ignore symptoms for too long.
Others worry about every small change.

The men who do best follow a different path.

They stay informed.
They ask questions.
They act when needed.
And they continue to live their lives fully.

Doctor's Pearl

You do not need perfect decisions. You need timely, thoughtful decisions.

Chapter Summary

- Most urinary symptoms are manageable and should not be ignored
- PSA is useful but must be interpreted carefully
- Not all prostate cancers require immediate treatment
- Treatment decisions should be individualized
- Lifestyle plays an important role in overall health
- Balanced awareness leads to better long-term outcomes

Final Action Plan

- Pay attention to your body and its signals
- Do not ignore persistent symptoms
- Avoid unnecessary fear or panic
- Maintain regular follow-up with your doctor
- Follow simple, healthy lifestyle habits
- Make decisions based on understanding, not emotion
- Stay positive and proactive

Final Message

Your prostate is a small gland, but it can have a meaningful impact on your life.

The reassuring truth is this.

Most prostate problems are manageable. Many are not dangerous. Even serious conditions can often be treated effectively when addressed at the right time.

You now have the knowledge to understand your body better.

Use it with confidence.

Take care of your health. Stay informed. And move forward with clarity, balance, and peace of mind.

APPENDIX 1: A Simple Self-Assessment for Your Urinary Symptoms

Why This Matters

Many men are unsure whether their symptoms are mild, moderate, or something that needs attention.

This simple self-check helps you understand where you stand.

Answer the following questions based on your experience over the past few weeks.

Your Symptoms

How often do you experience:

- A weak urine stream?
- Difficulty starting urination?
- Stopping and starting while urinating?
- A feeling that your bladder is not fully empty?
- Urgency to urinate?
- Frequent urination during the day?
- Waking up at night to urinate?

How to Think About Your Answers

- **Occasional, mild symptoms**
  Usually not urgent, but should be observed.
- **Frequent or bothersome symptoms**
  Should be discussed with your doctor.
- **Symptoms affecting sleep or daily life**
  Need proper evaluation and possible treatment.

Doctor's Note

This is not a diagnostic tool. It is a guide to help you recognize when it is time to act.

APPENDIX 2: Preparing for Your Doctor Visit – Make It Productive

Why Preparation Helps

A well-prepared visit saves time, reduces confusion, and leads to better decisions.

Many important details are forgotten during the visit unless you prepare in advance.

Before Your Visit

Make a simple note of:

- Your main symptoms
- When they started
- How often they occur
- Any recent changes
- Medications you are taking
- Previous PSA results, if available

Questions You Should Ask

- What is the most likely cause of my symptoms?

- Do I need any tests?
- What are my treatment options?
- What happens if I do nothing for now?
- What side effects should I expect?

During the Visit

- Speak openly and honestly
- Do not feel embarrassed
- Ask for clarification if something is unclear

Doctor's Note

A good consultation is a conversation, not a one-sided discussion.

APPENDIX 3: Daily Habits That Support Prostate Health

Small Steps That Add Up Over Time

These are simple habits that, when followed consistently, can improve symptoms and overall well-being.

Daily Routine Checklist

- Drink most fluids during the day, not late evening
- Limit caffeine and alcohol, especially at night
- Stay physically active
- Maintain a healthy weight
- Avoid constipation
- Follow a regular sleep schedule

Weekly Habits

- Review your symptoms
- Adjust habits if needed
- Stay consistent with exercise

Long-Term Habits

- Regular medical checkups
- PSA testing when appropriate
- Continued awareness of your body

Doctor's Note

There is no single powerful change. The real benefit comes from consistent, small improvements.

APPENDIX 4: When to Seek Immediate Medical Attention

Do Not Delay in These Situations

Most prostate symptoms develop slowly and can be managed calmly.

But certain symptoms require prompt medical attention.

Seek Immediate Care If You Have:

- Sudden inability to pass urine
- Severe pain with urination
- Fever with urinary symptoms
- Blood in urine
- Severe lower back or pelvic pain
- Unexplained weight loss

Why This Is Important

These symptoms may indicate:

- Infection
- Urinary retention
- More serious underlying conditions

Early action prevents complications.

Doctor's Note

Do not try to manage these symptoms at home. Prompt evaluation is important.

Thank You and Please Review the Book

Thank you for taking the time to read this book. I sincerely hope it has helped you understand your health a little more clearly and has given you practical, everyday steps you can follow with confidence. If you found this book helpful, **I would truly appreciate it if you could leave a brief and honest review.** Even a few lines sharing your experience can make a meaningful difference. Your feedback helps other readers find reliable, trustworthy health information and supports them in making better decisions for themselves and their families.

Warm regards,

Dr Prabhat Das

Continue your Healthcare Journey with these Books

Good health is a journey, not a single step. It is not achieved in one day or with one book. That is why I created the "Better Health with Dr Das Series", with each book addressing a different common condition. If you would like easy, practical guidance on other everyday health concerns, you may wish to explore the rest of books in this series.

Books in this series:

- Better Health starts Here: A Doctor's Guide to Staying Healthy After 40
- A Doctor's Easy Guide to Understanding & Managing OBESITY
- Doctor, What DIET Is Best for Me?
- Doctor, Why Can't I Lose Weight? A Doctor's Guide to Safe & Sustainable Weight Loss)
- A Doctor's Easy Guide to GLP-1 for Obesity
- A Doctor's Easy Guide to Understanding & Managing HIGH BLOOD PRESSURE
- A Doctor's Guide to Living Well With DIABETES
- A Doctor's Guide to Understanding & Managing THYROID DISEASES
- A Doctor's Guide to Understanding & Managing HIGH CHOLESTEROL
- A Doctor's Practical Guide to HEART HEALTH After 40: How to Protect Your Heart & Live Longer
- A Doctor's Guide to Healing & Reversing FATTY LIVER DISEASE: Simple, Natural & Science-Based Steps to Reduce Liver Fat and Prevent Complications

- Control Your ACID REFLUX, HEARTBURN & GERD: A Doctor's Practical Guide that Works
- Live Comfortably with IRRITABLE BOWEL SYNDROME: A Doctor's Practical Guide to Understanding & Managing IBS
- A Doctor's Practical Guide to Understanding & Managing GALLBLADDER STONES & OTHER PROBLEMS
- Take Control of COPD: A Doctor's Practical Guide to Better Breathing
- Living Better with ASTHMA: A Doctor's Practical Guide to Asthma Control
- SLEEP APNEA, INSOMNIA & OTHER SLEEP DISORDERS: A Doctor's Practical Guide to Better Sleep & Better Health
- Protect Your KIDNEYS: A Doctor's Practical Guide to Kidney Health & Prevention
- PROSTATE HEALTH: A Doctor's Practical Guide to Early Detection & Care
- ARTHRITIS: A Doctor's Practical Guide to Pain Control & Mobility
- A Doctor's Practical Guide to Fixing BACK PAIN Step by Step
- A Doctor's Practical Guide to Understanding & Managing GOUT & URIC ACID and Preventing Complications
- COMMON SKIN & HAIR PROBLEMS: A Doctor's Practical Guide to Skin & Hair Care
- DEMENTIA & MEMORY LOSS: A Doctor's Practical Guide to Prevention & Management
- Doctor, Why Am I TIRED All the Time? Fixing Fatigue & Getting Your Energy Back

9 781971 672557

Printed by Libri Plureos GmbH in Hamburg,
Germany